COMMUN
AS A CLIEN

ASSESSMENT
AND
DIAGNOSIS

COMMUNITY AS A CLIENT:
ASSESSMENT
AND
DIAGNOSIS

ZANA RAE HIGGS, R.N., Ed.D.

ASSOCIATE PROFESSOR
INTERCOLLEGIATE CENTER FOR NURSING EDUCATION
SPOKANE, WASHINGTON

DOROTHY DELL GUSTAFSON, R.N., M.S.N.Ed.

ASSISTANT PROFESSOR EMERITUS
INTERCOLLEGIATE CENTER FOR NURSING EDUCATION
SPOKANE, WASHINGTON

F. A. DAVIS COMPANY 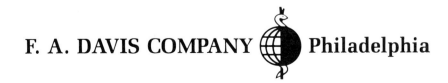 Philadelphia

Library of Congress Cataloging in Publication Data

Higgs, Zana Rae, 1940-
  Community as a client.

  Includes bibliographies and index.
  1. Community health nursing.   2. Community health nursing—Case studies.   I. Gustafson, Dorothy Dell, 1926-   . II. Title.
  RT98.H54   1985   610.73′43   84–21506
  ISBN 0 8036-4620-3

PREFACE

Our rapidly evolving society has produced a shift in the focus of the delivery of health care. Changes in population characteristics, life style, environmental factors, and health disorders have altered the leading causes of illness and death. On the one hand, there is an emphasis on highly sophisticated technology that saves lives. On the other hand, large groups of people need assistance to prevent and live with chronic health problems.

Constant assessment, reprioritization and planning of health care are necessary to predict and respond to these changes. For example, industrial health nurses are now as concerned with the body mechanics of workers who sit before a computer terminal for eight hours a day as they are with the effects of chemical and mechanical irritants. Although traditional efforts of working with individuals and their families remain an important aspect of health care, increasing emphasis has been placed on working with groups and with neighborhoods, communities, and whole regions to impact the health of their members. Nurses must play a vital role in these endeavors.

Nurses are well prepared to care for clients comprised of individuals and families. Emphasis has been placed on viewing the individual as a part of the family and community, and recognizing the impact of the family and community environment on the individual. The family is seen as a primary group with its own system of functioning and, as such, a focus for nursing care. The validity of viewing the community as a client has been supported by the statements of the American Nurses' Association and the American Public Health Association, which indicate that the community is the core focus of the community health nurse's practice. Therefore, community assessment is a fundamental skill required of community health nurses.

Since it is the responsibility of baccalaureate nursing programs to prepare staff level community health nurses, community assessment is currently being taught in varying degrees in baccalaureate nursing programs. Some programs focus on exploring and identifying the health needs of the community client. In other programs the community is assessed only as a support system for individuals or families receiving home health services.

There has been a lack of emphasis in the community health nursing texts on this important aspect of community health nursing practice. Although most texts accept the ANA definition of community health nursing and recognize the community as a client, major weaknesses exist in providing direction on how to assess and work with this client. For years this concern was shared with the book company detail men who came to our school to review their upcoming new books. Their persistent response echoed in our ears—"If you want it, write it." This book is a result of that advice and of a firm belief that the changes rapidly occurring in health care make it even more important that nurses are able to perform community assessments.

The intent of this book is to provide the baccalaureate nursing student and community health professionals with a resource which can be used to perform community assessments. The focus is on the application of the assessment phase of the nursing process to the community client. It is not our intent to provide a complete review of the literature of all disciplines which have contributed to the development of community assessments, but rather to cull out for the student those concepts and theories which can effectively be applied to nursing practice. The student is assisted to conceptualize the community as a client. A variety of approaches is provided from which the student may select a format to use in performing a community assessment.

Unit 1 provides a conceptual foundation for community health nursing and for the recognition of the community as a client. Unit 2 discusses conceptual approaches to community assessment. Four approaches were selected to discuss in detail. A brief review of other tools and approaches found in current literature is included. It is hoped this will encourage the reader to investigate methods of assessment which can be adapted for his or her use. Unit 3 explores nursing judgments made during the assessment process concluding with community diagnoses. Units 4 and 5 provide examples of how nurses in practice have performed community assessments and an introduction to the application of nursing theory to community assessments.

ZRH
DDG

ACKNOWLEDGMENTS

We would like to acknowledge the enthusiastic support and encouragement of relatives, friends, colleagues, and students. We particularly value the working relationship we shared as co-authors, which made the writing of this book an enjoyable experience.

ZRH
DDG

CONTRIBUTORS

CAROL ALLEN, R.N., M.S.
Assistant Professor
Intercollegiate Center for Nursing Education
Spokane, Washington

TINA BAYNE, R.N., M.S.
Assistant Professor
Intercollegiate Center for Nursing Education
Spokane, Washington

LAVONNE BERENTSON, R.N., M.S.N.
Assistant Professor
Nursing Advisor, Washington State University
Pullman, Washington

KATHERINE HILL CHAVIGNY, R.N., Ph.D., F.A.C.E.
Director, Office of Related Health Professions
American Medical Association
Chicago, Illinois

EDITH P. COLEMAN, R.N., M.S.
Crippled Children's Services Coordinator
Spokane County Health District
Spokane, Washington

LINDA FELVER, R.N., M.A.
Associate Professor
Intercollegiate Center for Nursing Education
Spokane, Washington

DONNA B. HAW, R.N., B.S.N.
Staff Nurse
Oregon Health Sciences University
Portland, Oregon

SHERRY BENNETT HOWARD, R.N., M.S.
Executive Director of Inpatient Nursing
Holy Family Hospital
Spokane, Washington

JO MCNEIL, R.N., M.N.
Occupational Health Specialist
Seattle–King County Health Department
Seattle, Washington

SHEILA L. MASTELLER, R.N., M.S.
Director of Clinical Services
Spokane Visiting Nurses Association
Spokane, Washington

CONTENTS

xii

INTRODUCTION TO COMMUNITY ASSESSMENT

The concept of community as a client is inherent in community health nursing practice. The bases for this perspective and discussion of descriptive characteristics of this client are the major thrusts of this unit. Assessment, as the initial step of the nursing process, forms the foundation for determining a client's health concerns regardless of whether the client is an individual, a family, or a community. However, the content of the assessment data, its sources, and techniques of collection vary. Emphasis is placed on that content and those sources and techniques relevant to community assessment.

CHAPTER 1

THE CONCEPT OF COMMUNITY AS A CLIENT

OBJECTIVES

THE LEARNER WILL

1. identify the relationship between the disciplines of nursing and public health in defining community health nursing.

2. differentiate between community health nursing practice and hospital nursing practice.

3. state the purpose for viewing the community as a client.

4. recognize the elements which describe a community.

5. list the functions of a community.

6. identify commonalities between the assessment of an individual and of a community.

Conceptualization of the community as a client and assessment of this client in order to identify health needs is a function of community health nursing practice. In order to understand this specific scope of practice it is important to have an understanding of the two major disciplines from which the community nurse draws knowledge, skills, and a conceptual approach to practice. These two disciplines are nursing and public health. It is through the integration of these two disciplines that the nurse defines the scope, attitudes, and activities of community health nursing practice.

PROFESSIONAL NURSING PRACTICE

In the introduction to the American Nurses' Association (ANA) *Standards of Nursing Practice*, nursing practice is defined as "a direct service, goal directed and adaptable to the needs of the individual, family and community during health and illness."[1] Nursing is a human service. Human beings are both its focus and the recipients of its activities. This focus is often referred to in statements that nursing is client- or patient-centered. Nursing is concerned with identification of health-related needs of people whether as individuals, families, or larger groups. Human beings, regardless of age or setting, are the recipients of nursing care that has as its goals the promotion, maintenance, and restoration of wellness, the prevention of illness, and care and support through illness and/or the dying process.

The concept "unit of service" or "unit of care" is used to refer to the focal point of a nurse's practice and thereby defines the client(s) served. The focus may be an individual, as in clinical nursing or clinical medicine; a family, as in family practice or family therapy; or a specifically defined group or community, as in community health nursing and public health practice. Each unit of service (patient/client) is viewed holistically as an individual entity interacting with its internal and external environments. The nurse is also concerned with the interrelationships among these units of service.

It is nursing's responsibility to identify and assure that the client's needs for help are met. Nurses utilize not only their own resources but also those of others, including the client. Therefore, the nurse has a major responsibility to coordinate, collaborate, and consult with the client, significant others within the client's support system, and other members of an interdisciplinary team in order to provide health care. In this process, the nurse must recognize and support the rights of clients to have differing needs, characteristics, values, cultural orientations, and systems of perceiving and responding to health needs.

Nursing care is implemented through use of the nursing process, which is a systematic, organized, continuous, cyclical series of interdependent steps that include client assessment, formulation of nursing diagnoses, planning and implementing nursing interventions, and evaluating change in the client's health status.

The nurse utilizes interventions such as health education, problem solving, and contracting to assist clients to develop their capabilities in meeting their own health needs. It may be said that the primary long-range goal of a nurse in relation to a client is to help that client reach an optimum level of wellness and become independent of the nurse. The nurse assists the client and the client's support system to become as totally responsible for fulfilling health needs as possible.

In order to accomplish its goals, nurses frequently must serve as a liaison between the client and the health care system—assisting the client to utilize resources, and influencing services to increase their usability. This process leads to identification, initiation, and support of needed improvements in health, nursing care, and the health care system.

The holistic, client-centered approach to health care with its focus on optimum wellness gives nurses a special perspective. This perspective is critical in planning for optimum health at all levels, from local to international. Therefore, it is important that nurses be involved with other health professionals and consumers in the process of assessing health needs and planning for health care.

In 1958, the revised National League for Nursing (NLN) accreditation standards determined that the League would no longer accredit educational programs that provide specialization at the baccalaureate level. At that time, the specialties of community health nursing and nursing education were majors in post-basic programs offered at the baccalaureate degree level. After five years, only those baccalaureate programs that included public health nursing would be accredited.[2] This directive mandated the responsibility for community health nursing preparation to baccalaureate nursing education. Therefore, it has become the responsibility of baccalaureate nursing education to prepare graduates who can 1) function in structured and unstructured settings, 2) function in a staff level position in community health agencies, and 3) identify health problems of a group of clients and populations at risk.

PUBLIC HEALTH PRACTICE

The purpose and goals of disciplines that provide service to the public are similar. They vary in their methods and scope of practice. Community health nursing draws heavily upon the science of public health.

Hilleboe defines public health as "the science and art of applying knowledge and skills from medicine and allied sciences in an organized community effort to maintain and improve the health of groups of individuals."[3] Hanlon states that Winslow's definition of public health written in 1920 continues to be the most widely accepted definition, which in part states: "Public Health is the science and art of 1) preventing disease, 2) prolonging life, and 3) promoting health and efficiency through organized community effort . . . so organizing those benefits as to enable every citizen to realize his birthrights of health and longevity."[4]

Hilleboe[5] also states that the practice of public health is conducted primarily on a public-health-physician–to–community basis rather than on a physician–to–individual-patient basis. Although there may be duplication in functions carried out by a public health physician and a physician in private practice, the major focus and responsibility of the public health physician is to the community as a whole. Although both physicians advocate measles immunizations, the public health physician may be concerned with preventing an outbreak of measles in the community. The physician in practice is concerned with protecting an individual client from contracting measles. Hilleboe clearly defines the intent of such practice when he delineates the objectives of public health: "to reduce the prevalence, incidence, mortality and debility from diseases and disabilities and to promote the general health of people."[6] Therefore, the focus of this practice is on the community as an entity, with emphasis on prevention and health promotion. The methods and resources used and priorities selected vary with each community and are based on an assessment of that community.

COMMUNITY HEALTH NURSING PRACTICE

Statements from the American Nurses' Association, Division of Community Health Nursing Practice, and the Public Health Nursing Section of the American Public Health Association clarify the relationship between these two disciplines.
    The ANA's definition of community health nursing states:

> Community Health Nursing is a synthesis of nursing practice and public health practice applied to promoting and preserving the health of populations. The nature of this practice is general and comprehensive. It is not limited to a particular age or diagnostic group. It is continuing, not episodic. The dominant responsibility is to the population as a whole. Therefore, nursing directed to individuals, families or groups contributes to the health of the total population. Health promotion, health maintenance, health education, coordination and continuity of care are utilized in a holistic approach to the family, group and community. The nurses' actions acknowledge the need for comprehensive health planning, recognize the influences of social and ecological issues, give attention to populations at risk and utilize the dynamic forces which influence change.[7]

This definition is consistent with the Nursing Section of the American Public Health Association's statements that

> The health and health care needs of a population are assessed by nurses or in collaboration with other disciplines. . . . The speciality of public health nursing is professional nursing directed toward a total community or population. . . . Its practice includes identification of subgroups and the families and individuals who comprise them. Emphasis is on planning for a community as a whole rather than on individual health care. Its purpose—to improve the health of the community through nursing intervention—is

achieved by working with and through community leaders, health-related groups, groups at risk, families and individuals and by becoming involved in relevant social action. . . . [One] distinguishing component of public health practice [is] community analysis.[8]

It is recognized that community health nurses are traditionally family oriented. The nurse works with the family as a client as well as the individuals within that family. Furthermore, the nurse is responsible for the health of all members of a family or household regardless of the initial referral or identified person whose health concerns lead to the first contact. For an individual living alone, the nurse perceives that person and those significant others who make up that person's support system as a family unit. Families are an integral part of a community. They are influenced by and contribute to the structure and functions of the community. In working with families, the nurse must analyze the impact of the community on the growth and development of the family.

Just as the nurse works with individuals within a family as well as the family as a client, the nurse also works with families within the community as well as the community as a client. For some, the concept of community as a client is foreign. Yet it is this concept and the concern of the nurse for the well being of this client that delineate the scope of community health nursing practice.

Recently, nursing has differentiated between the care provided in an acute care facility or an institution whose primary reason for existence is to provide care for people who are ill (episodic care) versus health care that is provided outside such a facility (distributive care). Additionally, episodic care refers to a time-bound "episode" in a person's life, related to the severity of the condition and requiring specialized services. Distributive care denotes a wide range of services provided to clients in the community over a period of time.

Health care transferred to a community setting with increased emphasis on primary care, nurse practitioner roles, and nurse clinics is not necessarily synonymous with community health nursing. Such practitioners may or may not regard the community within which they practice as a client. The main determinant to community health nursing practice is whether nursing is focused primarily on individuals and families, or whether it is also focused on and defined by the needs of the community.

The key focus of community health nursing practice, then, is on an identified population and provision of services that will directly or indirectly influence the well being of that community. Therefore, the nurse functioning in this scope of practice must always keep this perspective in mind—*that the community, as an entity, is a client.*

Although this may appear to be an insignificant difference, it is critical that a community health nurse "see the forest as well as the trees." Programs, services, and priorities may quickly become misdirected when the needs of the community as a whole shift. Great shifts in population characteristics can occur in a single geographic area over time, such as a deteriorating neighborhood with an increasing percentage of elderly population or the influx of immigrants into a specific area. If there is a focus only on the needs of individual clients, community health concerns are not addressed until they become problems, and then health care services are forced to use a crisis approach, redirecting resources (money, manpower, and services) in the classical "too little, too late" syndrome to respond to community health problems.

Community health nurses are also health oriented and as such place their major endeavors on preventive efforts: to promote health, to prevent illness, and to maintain the highest functioning level of the members of that community. With increasing longevity, chronic, long-term health disorders have surfaced as the conditions taking the heaviest toll on human life and suffering. Promoting, monitoring, and maintaining health take on a new perspective. New approaches directed to high-risk groups are being developed. Promoting healthy life styles becomes a key effort in preventing chronic illnesses, as does maintaining a healthful environment. Although changes in life style are undertaken by individuals, efforts to produce such changes and to improve the environment have been found effective when using a community-wide approach. A number of examples of such community-based programs may be found in *Healthy People*.[9] For example, in Milwaukee, in 1974, a community hypertension control program that involved health care organizations, industries, insurance companies, and local media screened and followed up on nearly 200,000 people. Over a period of four years, the heart attack rate in Milwaukee dropped 17 percent, and the stroke death rate dropped 38 percent.

If a nurse can develop and maintain the perspective that the community as a whole is the client, the nurse soon realizes that the community has a personality, a modus operandi or way of functioning. It has a historical perspective through which it has established a way of perceiving things, of coping with problems, and of making decisions. Changes in the community or attempts to maintain a sense of dynamic equilibrium are influenced by and influence surrounding communities. This type of understanding helps the nurse to approach the client holistically and to individualize care that will be effective in identifying and solving real or potential health problems. Given this scope of practice, it becomes critical that the nurse be able to assess, plan, and provide care to this unique client—the community.

THE COMMUNITY

In order to consider the idea of community as a client it is necessary to define the meaning of the term "community." There are as many variations in what may be termed community as there are differences in descriptions of individuals or families. A global definition of community that is precise, accurate, and comprehensive is difficult to formulate. There are, however, some key elements that characterize a community and identify it as a separate entity from its surrounding environment.

The following discussion of these key elements is based loosely on Connor's[10] list of components that comprise a community. All communities include individuals variously referred to as a group (of any size) or a social group (indicating some type of interaction). In relation to nursing and the human aspect of community, it can be simply stated that all communities include people. The people, as members of a social group, interact with each other formally and informally within some type of organizational structure. People who live in a particular resident hotel and workers who harvest crops are examples of communities with clearly defined and loosely defined structural boundaries, respectively.

The people in a community have a group perspective which differentiates them from other groups. This perspective or identity can take many forms or may be a combination of several characteristics. This includes an identity based on culture, beliefs, or mores. Examples of communities that fit this description based on ethnicity, race, or religion are black, Chicano, or Native American groups and Jewish or Catholic communities. When immigrants move from one country to another, they sometimes settle close to each other and form tightly knit groups with a common cultural identity. Many examples of this can be found in large metropolitan areas such as New York, Chicago, and Los Angeles, and in the agricultural areas of Pennsylvania and Minnesota.

Population aggregates, such as adolescents, emphysema victims, or any group whose members have a common characteristic, are sometimes used as an alternative in identifying a community for assessment purposes.[11] This is convenient for determining the group to be considered. It can also help in establishing a specific area of health needs on which to concentrate efforts. If the population aggregate does not function as an entity with a group identity and modes of interaction, implementation of a plan to resolve a health problem may involve working separately with each individual within the aggregate rather than with the entire group as a whole.

Some population aggregates have evolved into communities, such as the immigrants cited above or some elderly persons with their Gray Panther or other senior citizen organizations. Their common characteristics have contributed to the formulation of a cohesive group capable of group functioning.

Other common characteristics that encourage group identity are laws, occupation, or place of residence. For example, the United States has laws that differ from those of its neighboring countries, Mexico and Canada. Along with place of residence, these laws serve to identify its citizens as part of that country or community. Occupations also have identities and characteristics that can unite the participants into a sense of community.

When place of residence is used as one of the characteristics of a community, the term ''neighborhood'' is frequently used interchangeably with that of community. It is sometimes used to refer to a small community within a larger community structure. A neighborhood is a group of people residing in a specified area in the vicinity of each other. A neighborhood may or may not be a community. In order to be considered a community, this group of people must be a social group, have a group perspective, and function as a community.

There are innumerable examples to illustrate the idea of common characteristics. Whatever the basis for the commonality, the members of the group have a sense of being part of something and therefore have a group identity. Individuals identify with more than one group at the same time. They may belong to several communities or subcommunities simultaneously. This must be recognized as an influencing factor in their relationship within the community of interest. "This is similar to the way in which the human body consists of limbs and organs, each contributing something to the others and each dependent upon the rest for the health and efficiency of the whole man."[12] For example, the nurse is a member of the nursing community. As a voting citizen, the nurse is also a member of the political community, whether it be a ward, precinct, district, or state. The roles of nurse and voting citizen may influence each other but do not negate membership in either group.

The size of a community may vary from large to only a few members. Ecological problems are frequently viewed from a global community perspective. Air pollution affects the atmosphere surrounding the earth and all its inhabitants even though much of it is produced and must be corrected by the highly industrialized nations. At the other end of the size spectrum, individuals afflicted with a very rare disease may be few in number and still be classified as a community.

Spatial characteristics are commonly used to determine the boundaries of a community. Some definitions of a community include residence in a specific locality or geographic area.[13] This is quite easy to identify when the chosen community is a census tract, hospital, school, or apartment dwelling. The basis for initial identification of these communities has been a place of residence, identified structure, or geographic area used for a specific purpose. The people aspect of the community, so defined, then becomes those individuals interacting within the confines of these spatial characteristics.

If the community is designated by common characteristics of a particular group of people based on culture, beliefs, or customs, the task of delineating spatial characteristics becomes more difficult. Members of a group with a common identity do not always gather in a convenient cluster. Some may reside a great distance from the focus of interest. It may be realistic to create an artificial boundary to limit the size of a community to a workable unit that would still be representative of the community at large.

A group of baccalaureate students in a community health nursing class elected to identify the possible health problems of a particular ethnic population in the metropolitan area in which they were attending school. They had understood that this particular group lived in a single area on the north side of town. To their consternation, they discovered another segment of this particular ethnic group living across town on the south side. After discussions with representatives from both sides of town, they found that each group disapproved of the other's activities and life style. Neither group cared to be identified with the other.

The students wished to identify a specific geographic location for their community of study. They had to decide whether this was a single community group residing in two different locations or two specific communities with the same cultural background. One solution would have been to simply choose one or the other group as the community they wished to investigate. If this approach were used, they could not be sure that the data they collected represented the entire group. However, using both locations would make a concise geographic description more difficult.

Further investigation revealed common characteristics in both groups related to health problems and many similarities in relation to their strengths. Plans for change could be instituted in the same way for both groups. It was decided to consider both as a single community residing in two separate geographic locations.

A similar difficulty may present itself with the urban Native American community when a reservation is located nearby. Individuals may move back and forth between the two areas, resulting in a population that is always changing, but also one that may have dual residence affiliations.

Time is also an important dimension of the spatial characteristics of a community. Communities change and evolve over time as do the individual members of the community.

A person is spoken of as being homeokinetic—the term for the efforts of the body to maintain some kind of balance between wellness and illness so that it can function at its optimum level. A community might be said to be *communeokinetic*, that is, having the ability to adjust and to change to meet its needs so that it can function at its optimum level.

This ability to adjust is illustrated in the following example. A piece of farmland is sold to real estate developers who create a suburban housing area intended for young families. Babies are born and grow and the community changes to meet the needs—playgrounds, schools, sidewalks, traffic controls. These are all evidence of the *communeokinesis* of that particular community.

Each community also has variations in its periods of activity and inactivity similar to the biorhythms of humans. This can be dependent upon the culture or customs of the residents, climate, occupation, or a variety of other factors. Activity in Las Vegas is on quite a different schedule from that of an Iowa farming community. In order to identify activity patterns, it is important that assessment data be collected over a span of time.

Communities are social units with identifiable characteristics similar to those of an individual or family. They exist within a larger social environment or system. Interaction takes place among members of the community, between members and the surrounding system, and between the community and its environment. These relationships have to do with the management of the community. The community is governed by formal and informal rules and laws whose bases vary depending on the nature of the community. The community is organized and functions in order to meet the needs of its members.

Maslow[14] has identified a "hierarchy of needs" of individuals as a theoretical basis for motivation. These basic needs and their organization in hierarchical levels are a useful way of assessing an individual. Because the community is being viewed as an entity (the client), the idea of need for survival, growth, development, and fulfillment of a community is also applicable.

Community needs can be arranged in a hierarchical order that is consistent with that developed by Maslow. The same premise that the lower level needs must be met before the higher level needs can be addressed also holds true (Fig. 1-1).

In order for these needs to be satisfied, certain functions must be accomplished either by the individual members of the community, by the community as a whole, or by the surrounding larger society for the benefit of the community members. These functions are supported by laws, rules, and mores developed both inside and outside the community unit. Klein[15] has identified certain functions of a community that are necessary for its existence. These have been reorganized into seven areas that identify the functions of the community as a client. They include a system for

1. Utilization of space—housing, access and egress, socialization and recreation.
2. Means of livelihood—employment, sustenance, health.
3. Production, distribution, and consumption of goods and services.
4. Protection of its members—creating and enforcing norms and controls, prevention of physical disasters.
5. Education—socialization of adults, children, and newcomers, ongoing enrichment.
6. Participation—communication, social interaction, support.
7. Linkage with other systems providing for needs of its members when the community is unable or elects not to carry out its functions.

In summary, it can be said that a *community is a group of people with a common identity or perspective, occupying space during a given period of time, and func-*

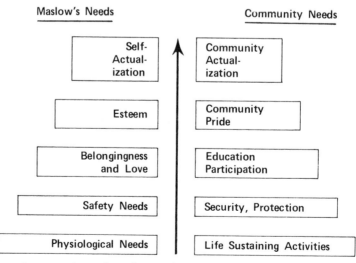

FIGURE 1-1. A comparison of Maslow's identification of basic needs of the individual with those of the community as a client.

tioning through a social system to meet its needs within a larger social environment.

COMPARISON OF NURSING ASSESSMENT OF AN INDIVIDUAL WITH THAT OF A COMMUNITY

Now that the client—community—has been defined and described, the nursing process can be used as a means of providing nursing care to this client. Just as one would not presume to give care to an individual without first assessing that person's needs, a community health nurse assesses the community in order to identify needs, establish priorities, plan, implement, and evaluate care. Assessment of a community uses many of the same skills and data bases that nurses use to assess individual clients; however, the content of the assessment data is different. The following are examples of some of the assessment skills and resultant data that a nurse uses in assessing an individual client and how these relate to assessing a community.

Observation/Inspection

In making observations of individual clients, the nurse uses the senses of sight, sound, smell, and touch. What does the wound look like? Is the area around it warm to touch? What kind and amount of drainage is there? What does the drainage smell like? What does the baby's cry sound like? Is it high pitched?

These same senses are used in observing a community. What does the nurse see? What do the people, the geography, and the environment look like? What sounds can one hear? Is it noisy or quiet? What languages are spoken? Can industries be identified by their sounds in the community? What foods are cooking? Are flower gardens in bloom? Is the air polluted, such as by fumes from pulp mills? What food preferences are in local restaurants or neighborhood stores? In a community, the sense of touch may be more of a sense of feel, that is, the feeling one gets of a community. Is it warm, open and friendly, or hostile and distrustful of strangers?

Vital Signs (Auscultation, Palpation, Percussion)

The nurse uses these skills to determine and describe the functioning of vital systems. What is the blood pressure? Are the lung fields clear? Are peripheral pulses palpable? Can one differentiate between the borders of the liver and fluid in the abdomen by percussion?

In a community, such vital information takes the form of biostatistics that describe the health status of the community. What are the demographic data that describe the population and the vital statistics, such as births and deaths? What epidemiological data indicate the occurrence and distribution of health problems in the population?

Laboratory Values

These assist the nurse to verify impressions from the assessment or give direction for additional assessment. What organism is cultured from that wound? What is the individual client's hemoglobin, arterial blood gases, blood glucose level?

In the community, the nurse may need to be able to monitor and certainly to interpret many aspects of environmental data. What is the carbon monoxide level? The noise level? What is the cause of an epidemic of nausea and vomiting? Is the water supply contaminated by sewage?

Nursing History/Interview

What is the individual thinking and feeling? What are the perceived health problems, ability to cope, and need for service? What are significant others' impressions of the client's situation? What resources and support system does the client use or have available to deal with health problems?

Just as the nurse collects subjective data—for example, the client's perspective, beliefs, values, perceived needs, and goals—the nurse assessing a community determines what the community sees as its concerns and needs. What attitudes do they have toward health? What history of health problems? What is the population's perspective of life, culture, values, and beliefs within the community? These psychosocial, cultural-anthropological data are extremely important in determining priorities and appropriateness of alternative interventions. What community resources (facilities, money, manpower) are available and used to meet community needs? In order to have an impact on the community, the nurse must assess and develop an understanding of the social–political-power (decision-making) system within the community. It is as important to understand how a community works or "what makes it tick" as it is with an individual client.

Clinical Judgment

For the individual client, the nurse must know the meaning of the data and interpret their significance. Is the client's behavior a result of the disease process, a drug response, or anxiety? Is this blood pressure within normal limits for the client's age? The data must be compared with age- and sex-specific "norms" or standards of acceptable ranges.

The nurse assessing a community compares assessment data with norms and standards. Is the air quality within acceptable limits? Is the infant mortality rate higher than the national average? Do changes in data over time indicate that the health status of the community is getting "better" or "worse"? Is availability of services matching shifts in populations—young to old, rural to urban? What are the community's strengths as well as its limitations? What is the developmental status of the community? Is it growing or declining? How well is the community able to provide for the basic needs of its population?

Such an assessment is consistent with that described in Standard I of the ANA Standards of Nursing Practice. In summary, the standard states that health status data include growth and development; biophysical status; emotional status; cultural, religious, and socioeconomic background; performance of activities of daily living; patterns of coping; interaction patterns; client's perception of and satisfaction with his or her health status; client's health goals; environment (physical, social, emotional, ecological); available and accessible human and material resources. These data are collected from client/patient, family, significant others, health care personnel, individuals within the immediate environment, and/or the community. Data are obtained by interview, examination, observation, and reading records and reports.[16]

In summary, one aspect of professional nursing practice is community health nursing. A primary concern of the community health nurse is the community client. Assessment as the first stage of the nursing process can be applied to this client.

REFERENCES

1. EXECUTIVE COMMITTEE AND STANDARDS COMMITTEE OF AMERICAN NURSES ASSOCIATION: *Standards of Nursing Practice.* American Nurses Association, Kansas City, Missouri, 1973, p 1.

2. TINKHAM, C AND VOORHIES, E: *Community Health Nursing: Evolution and Process.* Appleton-Century-Crofts, New York, 1972, p 83.

3. HILLEBOE, H AND LARIMORE, G: *Preventive Medicine.* WB Saunders, Philadelphia, 1966, p 3.

4. HANLON, J AND PICKETT, G: *Public Health Administration and Practice.* CV Mosby, St Louis, 1979, p 4.

5. HILLEBOE, *op cit,* p 7.

6. Ibid, p 8.

7. EXECUTIVE COMMITTEE AND STANDARDS COMMITTEE OF AMERICAN NURSES ASSOCIATION, DIVISION ON COMMUNITY HEALTH NURSING PRACTICE: *Standards of Community Health Nursing Practice.* American Nurses Association, Kansas City, Missouri, 1974, p 1.

8. PUBLIC HEALTH NURSING SECTION, AMERICAN PUBLIC HEALTH ASSOCIATION: *The Definition and Role of Public Health Nursing in the Delivery of Health Care.* The American Public Health Association, Washington, DC, 1980.

9. US DEPARTMENT OF HEALTH, EDUCATION AND WELFARE: *Healthy People.* The

Surgeon General's Report on Health Promotion and Disease Prevention. PHS Publication #79-550717, Washington, DC, 1979, pp 99, 119, 121.

10. CONNOR, DM: *Understanding Your Community*, ed 2. Development Press, Ottawa, Canada, 1969.

11. KURTZMAN, C, ET AL: *Nursing process at the aggregate level. Nursing Outlook*, December 1980, pp 737–739.

12. CONNOR, *op cit*, p 7.

13. FROMER, MJ: *Community Health Care and the Nursing Process*. CV Mosby, St Louis, 1979, p 166.

14. MASLOW, AH: *Motivation and Personality*, ed 2. Harper & Row, New York, 1970, pp 35–47.

15. KLEIN, DC: *Community Dynamics and Mental Health*. John Wiley & Sons, New York, 1968, p 7.

16. EXECUTIVE COMMITTEE AND STANDARDS COMMITTEE OF AMERICAN NURSES ASSOCIATION: *Standards of Nursing Practice*. American Nurses Association, Kansas City, Missouri, 1973.

CHAPTER 2

SOURCES AND TECHNIQUES
OF ASSESSMENT

OBJECTIVES

THE LEARNER WILL

1. define community assessment.

2. identify five purposes for community assessment.

3. recognize factors that affect the focus of a community assessment.

4. given a specific problem situation,

    a. identify the appropriate technique(s) for assessment.

    b. list possible sources of information.

    c. recall strengths and limitations of the chosen technique(s).

DEFINITION OF COMMUNITY ASSESSMENT

Community assessment is the initial step in the problem-solving process used to promote the health of a community. Blum[1] describes the assessment of a community as the application of a measuring tool or assortment of tools to a defined social area and applying judgment to the data gathered to determine priorities for program planning and evaluation. Planning and implementation should not proceed until there has been a comprehensive collection and analysis of the factors that contribute to health disorders and those that assist in the maintenance of health. A firm and accurate foundation forming the basis for the next steps in the process gives direction to the investigator. Assessment may be divided into three major components: the systematic collection of information or data, the organization of those data in such a manner that interrelationships may be determined, and the analysis or interpretation of the data resulting in formulation of conclusions. In nursing, these conclusions are referred to as nursing diagnoses.

The factors that must be assessed relate to the description of a community—a group of people, the space they occupy, and how they function and relate to one another and the larger society. Within this context, the concept of health disorders has a much broader perspective than simply that of disease. Physiological, sociocultural, psychological, and spiritual considerations all influence the health of a community.

PURPOSE OF COMMUNITY ASSESSMENT

The purpose of an assessment determines the type of data to be collected and the assessment techniques to be used. There are various reasons for performing a community assessment. Initiation of an assessment is based on one or a combination of the following purposes.

Needs Identification

A community assessment to identify health needs should be performed on an ongoing basis by those responsible for providing health care to the community. When the community is unknown to the health care worker, it is important to determine the existing needs as soon as possible. For example, the community health nurse assigned the responsibility for a new area would begin immediately to note the nature of the population being served, the health problems that may be encountered, and previous services provided before program activities can be planned and prioritized.

The nurse starts with a comprehensive community assessment, making a particular effort to avoid prejudgment of the community. Preconceived ideas of the health problems may mislead the investigation, waste time and energy, or result in overlooking other health concerns. It is important to obtain the clients' perspectives of their health needs. An objective assessment leads to problem identification and may be likened to a routine health assessment or holistic health screening assessment of an individual.

Problem Clarification

Frequently, the reason for being assigned to a community or choosing to concentrate efforts in a community is that a particular problem has been presented as a health concern. It is necessary to understand the specific nature and magnitude of the problem as well as its relationship to the community and the environment. The data collected are focused on determining factors related to the specific problem. For example, an annual increase in the incidence of measles in a certain census tract may indicate a resident population with a low percentage of individuals immunized against the disease. However, if it were discovered that the permanent population has a high rate of immunization but that a migrant population that moves into the community seasonally has contributed to the increased incidence of the disease, the timing, location, and direction of efforts to eradicate the disease would be very different.

Problem clarification may be likened to a chief-complaint–oriented history and assessment of an individual client. In this type of assessment, the focus is on an already identified problem rather than prevention or early detection of developing problems.

Desire Analysis

Representatives of a community may request resolution of a specific problem within their area or group. It is important to be aware of community concerns. These concerns may be similar to already identified health needs and may provide helpful additional data. Those expressing the desire may not represent the opinions of the entire community. The nature of the problem, the setting, possible interventions and priorities in relation to existing resources, programs, and funding must all be investigated. It is important to be aware of any differences in values held by consumers and providers of health care. For example, a delegation of rural residents whose well water has recently shown an increase in chemical contaminants may approach the environmental section of the local health department with their problem. Areas that can be assessed include the nature of the chemical and its effects; the extent of contamination; its source and route of progress through the water system; the standards, rules, and regulations governing controls in this situation; and any other resources available to the well owners or health department to deal with these concerns. Planning and priority setting would depend upon the outcome of the findings of the assessment.

Resource Identification

Implementation of plans for resolution of a health problem does not always involve the initiation of new programs. Every community has resources that are used by the residents for their individual benefit. Listing the available resources and determining methods of sharing their availability are sometimes the only steps necessary for solution of a particular problem. Supplements to or extensions of existing programs may be a much more economical approach than investing monies in an additional program. Duplication of resources is most common in a community in which there is a lack of communication among agencies.

Resource Utilization

Closely related to identification of resources is an assessment of their use by the people for whom they were intended. There may be many reasons for lack of utilization related to values, income, and customs of the individual clients along with accessibility and availability of the resource. Becker[2] indicates that an individual's decision to use resources is based on an estimate of benefits minus cost, with cost referring to many factors, including time and energy. These elements need to be carefully assessed and considered. The staff of a family planning agency in a small rural community was distressed over the lack of utilization of their resource by the residents in an area in which the need had been clearly identified. An outside consultant quickly noticed that the entrance to the agency was located on the main street across from a cafe that was the local gathering place. Questioning potential users of this service indicated that no one was willing to enter through the all-too-public entrance and risk being recognized in this small community. Moving the agency office to a multi-use building increased utilization drastically.

FOCUS OF ASSESSMENT

Numerous factors affect the focus of a community assessment and the range of activities involved in this process. The assessment may be limited to observations and review of existing, readily available information or may entail designing and implementing a complex research study. A nurse who cares for a hospitalized patient for the first time after morning report initiates that care on a brief assessment and continues the assessment process concurrent with providing direct nursing care. Likewise, a community health nurse who is new to a community begins to practice community health nursing prior to performing a thorough community assessment. The nurse continuously assesses the community to form a basis for practice.

The focus and complexity of the assessment to be performed will be affected by 1) the purpose of the assessment, 2) the conceptual approach(es) chosen in designing the assessment, 3) the size of the community to be assessed, 4) the time available to perform the assessment, 5) the expertise of those participating in the assessment, 6) the relationship between cost and benefit of the assessment, and 7) the political environment within the community. If a community is experiencing an outbreak of infectious hepatitis, the assessment will be narrowly focused on identifying the source of the disease and its transmission, followed by quick intervention to interrupt the further transmission of the disease. It may be only after this intervention that a comprehensive picture of the total outbreak is determined so that steps can be taken to prevent future occurrences.

TECHNIQUES USED IN COMMUNITY ASSESSMENT

There are various techniques that are useful in performing a community assessment. A number of techniques should be used in assessing a community. The conceptual model chosen for the assessment and the purpose of the assessment provide direction in selection of appropriate techniques.

Epidemiological Data Analysis*

Epidemiological data analysis refers to an assessment of the occurrence and distribution of health disorders in a population. This approach uses two major types of information—vital statistics and morbidity statistics. Vital statistics refer to data collected from the registration of births, deaths, marriages, and divorces. This registration is required by state law. Some form of statistics regarding deaths has been kept in New York City since the late 1800s. Since then, states have developed various laws regarding registration of vital statistics. By 1933, each state had birth/death registration. States have delegated the responsibility for collecting the data to the local registrar. This information is forwarded to a designated state office and then to the National Center for Health Statistics at the Center for Disease Control in Atlanta, Georgia. After the data are collected and analyzed, the results are distributed to state and local agencies for their information. These data are used for need identification, program planning, and research studies.

Birth certificate information usually includes race, education, and ages of parents, mother's previous pregnancies and their results, infant's birth weight, prenatal care, whether or not this was a multiple birth, complications of pregnancy and delivery, injury or malformation of infant, and whether birth occurred at home or in the hospital. There is also a special form to report fetal death. Death certificates are the major source of mortality statistics and generally include place of residence, place of occurrence, age, sex, race, national origin, cause of death, contributing causes, and other existing conditions not related to cause of death. Causes and conditions are coded according to the International Classification of Diseases system.

---

*For a detailed description of this approach, see Chapter 3.

Data from birth, death and fetal death certificates may be obtained from local and state health departments. Data formats and how soon data are available vary from community to community. For example, data may be provided in a computer printout by month that lists data from each certificate. The information may be summarized by census tract or county. The information may be already calculated into rates. A rate is:

$$\frac{\text{Number of cases occurring}}{\text{Total of population at risk of developing the condition}} \times \begin{array}{c} \text{constant} \\ \text{(e.g., 10,000)} \end{array}$$

If the data have not been calculated into rates, the nurse who wishes to compare one area with another must calculate rates based on an estimate of the population in the area under study. Local health departments usually have population estimates and formulas from which rates can be calculated. Each state publishes an annual report of health data drawn from these certificates. The National Center for Health Statistics, Division of Vital Statistics annually publishes *Vital Statistics in the United States*,[3] which provides national statistics as well as those for states and some metropolitan areas. These volumes are available at any library that serves as a repository for government documents. It takes about three years for the most recent data to be available in published form. Similar international information is available from the World Health Organization and Pan American Health Organization.

The information related to death is known as *mortality data*. These data are useful in determining the number of deaths in a given population according to cause, the previously mentioned characteristics of the deceased, and the interaction among these factors. Mortality data are relatively accurate and well reported. They clearly identify who is dying of what reported conditions.

There are certain limitations to mortality data. First, because it is controlled by state law, information regarding characteristics of the deceased varies from state to state. Only one cause of death may be designated on the death certificate. An adequate way of identifying the relationships of multiple causes in classifying deaths has not been developed. For example, the death certificate for a person with congestive heart failure who dies from pneumonia may list pneumonia as the cause of death and congestive heart failure as a contributing cause. Also, the physician may choose to indicate a more socially acceptable condition as the cause of death, for example, heart failure rather than third-stage syphilis. The report may list the condition that caused death, but not the contributing factors. For example, smoking may have been the major contributing factor implicated in the development of lung cancer, which is the reported cause of death. Comparisons of death rates or mortality among different populations have certain limitations. Unless rates are age-adjusted, comparisons among populations with different percentages of age groups can be misleading. In a small population, a single death may increase the death rate from that disease by 100 percent. Yet, depending upon the condition, this may be insignificant. Inasmuch as the classification categories defined by the International Classification of Disease are reviewed and revised every 10 years, comparing death rates over time may be misleading because diseases may be newly identified or reclassified. Finally, such data tell relatively nothing about the well being of those living in the community.

Epidemiological data also include *morbidity data.* These data refer to the number of cases of a health disorder in a population. There are three major sources of such information. First, certain communicable diseases are required by law to be reported to the health department. Two conditions that are also required to be reported but for which the mechanism of transmission is still unclear are autoimmune deficiency syndrome (AIDS) and toxic shock syndrome. These data are available from local and state health departments and are reported in the *Morbidity and Mortality Weekly Report*[4] by the Center for Disease Control in Atlanta. Similar international information is available from the World Health Organization and Pan American Health Organization. Unfortunately, some of the reportable communicable diseases are under-reported. Thus, the number of reported cases of gonorrhea in the community, for example, is used to formulate an estimate of the incidence of that condition in the population rather than being taken as a true indication of the incidence. This is referred to as the "iceberg effect," with the reported cases representing the small but visible tip of the iceberg and the unreported cases representing the larger but invisible portion.

The second source is "self-reported" health disorders such as those determined by the National Health Survey. This survey was instituted in 1956 by the U.S. Public Health Service and includes data from a large sample of households scientifically chosen throughout the country. The results are published in a series of issues of *Vital and Health Statistics*[5] by the National Center for Health Statistics. Self-reporting in such surveys has been found to be valid, which means that reported conditions are consistent with clinical findings upon examination.

The third source of morbidity data is reports of clinical evidence. This type of data is often referred to as "rates under treatment" and is available from hospital records, clinic and physician records, mass screenings, and registers such as the Cancer Registry. Insurance companies also publish such data. Voluntary health agencies, such as the American Heart Association and the American Lung Association, are good sources of information regarding the specific disease(s) with which they are involved. Armed services, large industries, and prepaid health plans also compile morbidity statistics regarding those involved with the organization. Because of the confidentiality of records and the need to assure anonymity, these data may be difficult to obtain. However, once these rights are assured, this is a relatively inexpensive way of identifying health problems that are being treated and services that are being rendered in a community. Because it is unlikely that such data will be available from all public and private sources in the community, this approach provides only a sample of those who are obtaining services. Also, it is difficult to estimate the degree of need by focusing only on those served. Finally, such data continue to be oriented to describing already diagnosed diseases.

The nurse should be creative in identifying sources of such data. For example, if interested in the number of children under age 2 who have ingested poisonous substances, the Poison Control Center would be the agency to contact. If attempting to determine the degree to which rape is a problem in a community in which there is no rape crisis service, the police department and hospital emergency rooms might have such data. Again, there is no assurance that all cases are reported. The nurse may use agency records as a source of data to determine patterns or shifts in numbers of clients receiving services for various health disorders.

Demographic Data Analysis

Demographic data describe the population and can be used to determine changes in the characteristics of a population over time. These data are obtained according to census tract by the U.S. Bureau of Census every 10 years.[6] Census tracts are smaller divisions of a geographic area which provide for counting and describing populations. The census data include such information as age, sex, race, occupation, national origin, marital status, education, income, and information about dwellings (year built; rented or owned; value of property; number of rooms; number of people per room).

City, county, and regional planning offices often have copies of this information plus periodic updated estimates. The census is published and usually available at the public library and health departments. Any governmental or university office involved in grant writing would have such data.

Demographic data are usually considered an indirect indicator of health concerns because of the association between these characteristics and health disorders which have been identified through epidemiological research. There has been established a strong relationship between the infant mortality (proportion of children dying before age 1) and the socioeconomic status of the community, such as income per capita, education (literacy), and sanitation. Demographic data are used to help determine which segments of the population are at risk of developing which health disorders and what services will be needed. For instance, a census tract which has a high proportion of pre-school-age children living in near poverty level income and substandard housing could be expected to have high risk infants and mothers and require related services.

One strength of demographic data analysis is the accessibility of the data. The data has already been tabulated and requires simple procedures such as calculating percents to convert the tabulated data into a meaningful form for comparisons among populations. Secondly, the information from a census is comprehensive because of the high proportion of the population returning the census questionnaire.

Because of the interaction between the people and the environment, demographic data should not be looked at in isolation. Health disorders are determined by the relationship between people and their environment.

Observations

Observations of a community are descriptive data gathered by health professionals using their *senses* as the data-gathering tools. This process may involve a single individual or a group of people. The data collected are a source of immediate information which can be useful in a variety of ways.

The nurse assigned to a new community client is rather like the community health nurse or social worker who is planning a first home visit to a family. One of the first decisions is whether the records on the family should be reviewed to ascertain the existing problems as perceived by previous health workers or should the records be reserved for later review and the first visit be one to gain a fresh perspective regarding the family situation. The opportunity for this happens only once in each new referral.

Observations can be used to develop tentative ideas regarding present or potential health concerns of the community. These hypotheses can be validated by other sources of data. Observations can also be used to verify or to negate previously identified health needs. They may also be useful by not only substantiating a health need but by gaining a different perspective on the situation.

The advantages of careful observations in a community are that they personalize the area for the worker. It is natural to have the need to mentally visualize the community before one can grasp the full import of the situation. Because each person will have a different view and emphasis regarding health problems, there will be as many new pieces or supportive pieces of data as there are individuals participating in the observational process.

Participants must remain as objective as possible in this subjective activity. Care must be taken to recognize that individuals have their own values and beliefs which must not be imposed upon others. Observations should be made over a period of time to validate impressions.

Environmental Indices

Each community exists within its own unique physical environment. In order to determine the needs of a community, a description of its environmental features and their relationship to some predetermined standards must be established. A comparison of these standards with existing conditions is sometimes called the *quality* of the environment.

An environmental description can be obtained by investigating natural conditions such as the topography, geography, climate, flora, fauna, and the orientation of the area in relation to the elements of wind, air, and water. Human habitation influences environmental resources. Information must also be obtained on the density of the population; amount, type, and use of structures; and living or industrial activities which result in a contribution to, depletion of, or pollution of the natural resources of the area.

Sources for descriptive information about the environment are maps, atlases, libraries, chambers of commerce, the weather bureau, local and state government agencies, agricultural departments, and universities who have an interest in environmental concerns. Local newspapers and legislative offices may be very helpful, particularly if there is a current concern regarding some aspect of the environment.

The federal government and some state and local authorities have established standards for environmental features such as air, water, noise, and sewage. The responsibility for monitoring and controlling these varies from community to community. Data resulting from environmental monitoring can be obtained from local health departments or the Environmental Protection Agency (EPA).

Accumulation of this type of information can be very helpful. It produces data which may initiate problem investigation or substantiate previously identified conditions within a community. In the Willamette Valley of Oregon, one of the major agricultural activities is growing grass seed for lawns. A common practice was to burn the stubble fields after harvest in late summer in order to clean up the fields and stimulate plant growth for the following year. Complaints about the smoke-filled air were common every burning season. Efforts to find alternative methods for the relatively inexpensive open field burning were not initiated until conclusive environmental data were gathered. These data showed the extent of the problem in terms of the amount of air pollution in relation to government standards, the large geographic area it covered because of topography and air currents, and the number of people it affected.

The value of such data is that it is objective. If it is comprehensive, it should be relatively free of bias. Its limitations include availability and accuracy. Monitors for air pollution, for example, might not be placed in locations that result in a precise determination of pollution levels in the entire area.

Key Informant Interviews

The concept of key informant refers to those individuals who have a "finger on the pulse" of a community. They are in a position to know the community's needs, the effectiveness of its current services, and the political structure within the community through which change can be channeled. Key informants are usually involved in the formal or informal communication and/or power structure within the community. They may be categorized into two types: they may be a part of the governmental, health or other community service agencies (both private and public), or they may be a part of the informal power structure in which they serve as key opinion makers. Many communities have individuals within them who may not currently hold any significant office or agency position within the community but whose opinion is highly valued and whose support may be crucial to establishment and success of a new program.

The key informant approach entails an interview of selected individuals, utilizing a consistent interview schedule to obtain consistency of data collected. Face-to-face interview versus phone or mailed questionnaire does provide the key informant the opportunity for a free exchange of ideas and provides a high response rate.

The nurse will need to work within a community for a while to be able to identify those who are significant informal community leaders. Observation of the problem-solving process used by a community and listening to community members' descriptions of the influence process in the community will help the nurse identify these people. A disadvantage of the approach is the lack of assurance that these individuals' opinions are representative of those of the people in the community. This is particularly true when the community includes a variety of ethnic, cultural, or socioeconomic groups. It is important that the nurse assures input from such major subgroups within a community. Views of key informants who hold governmental or agency positions in the community are affected by their educational preparation and their agency's perspective of community affairs, and so they may be viewed as "outsiders" of the community.

Community Forum Approach

The community forum approach uses a series of public meetings to obtain opinions of residents about the needs and services of the community. These may be open forums where everyone interested is invited to attend or may focus on specific groups in order to determine the special needs of the group. The community forum is a relatively inexpensive way of obtaining opinions of members of the community. It provides a different perspective than does the key informant approach, but those in attendance may not represent the opinions of the community as a whole either.

Factors affecting attendance include how well the forum is publicized, the degree to which such forums are normally used by a community to develop dialog between officials and members of that community, and the degree to which the topic under discussion is of interest or an issue in the community. It may be difficult to maintain the focus of the forum on the questions that the nurse wishes answered. It is important that the meetings do not heighten expectations that then cannot be met. A community forum may be viewed as a decision-making process or a commitment to desired interventions rather than an information-gathering process. The purpose of the forum must be made clear to the participants.

Opinion Surveys

An opinion survey is an approach to collect data from a sample of the population of a community regarding their opinions of the health needs and services in the community or information regarding their health and use of services. Such surveys usually are performed by door-to-door interviews, telephone interviews, or mailed questionnaires. This tends to be a more expensive method of gathering information than the key informant or community forum approaches. The expense is due to either the amount of staff time needed or the postage for initial and follow-up contacts. With relatively poor initial response to mailed questionnaires, additional effort is required to obtain a large enough number of completed questionnaires from individuals in the community to be able to assume that their opinions will be representative of the opinions of the remaining population not surveyed.[7]

Certain kinds of information are not likely to be shared through such an approach even though the respondent remains anonymous. If information from low income groups is desired, a telephone survey will likely reach a smaller proportion of this group. A mailed survey is not useful for groups who have low educational levels or for whom English is not the primary language. However, a well-designed survey provides the best information about individuals' perceptions of their needs and use of services. Babbie provides a thorough description of considerations for development of a survey.[8]

Sociomedical Health Indicators

Recently, efforts have been made to develop indicators of the health rather than the illness status of a population. These have focused on mental well being, social well being (extent to which an individual is able to fill social roles and tasks), personal life style, and health-related practices. A number of mental and social well being indices have been developed for elderly populations. Major risk reduction studies have been undertaken to determine the extent of health-related practices within populations that place members at risk of developing health disorders. For instance, smoking, drinking, exercise, stress, and isolation have been studied. This approach usually uses a mailed questionnaire. Sample questionnaires may be obtained from a number of sources for use or revision in local community studies. As with opinion surveys, this is a relatively expensive approach but provides relatively accurate data. It requires a large enough number of people responding to assure their answers on the questionnaire represent the remainder of the community not surveyed.

Historical Perspective

An understanding of the history of a community provides a background regarding its past development, values, attitudes, and systems of operation. This information can be found in libraries, museums, and newspaper files. Local historians or historical societies may also be helpful. Someone who may have a formally published history of the area might be willing to share additional private files. Some areas of the country are of relative recent development (20th century). Older residents may be able to provide interesting oral histories. A smaller community, such as an agency or business, may have its own historical records.

A historical perspective not only provides descriptive information on the development of the community but also identifies previous problems and successes or failures in solutions of these problems. It can identify a current health need as one that has been ongoing or newly acquired. It can also help project potential future problems and put identified problems in perspective. Because a community goes through developmental stages as do individuals and families, the historical perspective gives an understanding of the developmental process this community is experiencing.

The worth of this type of information is based upon the objectivity and accuracy of the source and an objective interpretation of the information. The investigator must be aware of values and beliefs of the population at the time being reported and avoid erroneous conclusions based on current values and beliefs.

Resource Analysis

Analysis of resources is based upon an identification and description of available assistance for the maintenance of health and resolution of health problems. The description should also include information on use of the resource by the population it intends to serve. The areas to be analyzed are drawn from both the structure and functions of a community. These can include government, finance and economy, education, recreation and entertainment, communication, transportation, public safety and legal assistance, community or professional organizations, and health care or human services.

In most communities the phone book, city directories, and local newspapers will give a quick initial overview of resources available. Individual agency or organizational representatives can supply more specific information and may be helpful in directing the investigator to further sources. An information and referral service or booklets listing health services may be available in some communities. Local telephone operators or librarians are sometimes most informative. Colleges or universities may be helpful, especially if part of their curriculum involves health concerns or preparation of health professionals.

Resources for alternate methods of health care should not be overlooked, particularly if the population includes a specific ethnic or cultural group differing from the group in power. These may be more difficult to identify because of lack of general acceptance by the established society. There may also be a lack of trust by the users of the alternate care methods toward the established health care providers which would make information difficult to obtain. The Chicano or Native American may use both health care systems but be willing to discuss only the one represented by the investigator.

The existence and use of resources is dependent upon societal attitudes or values and the power or decision-making process of the community. Key informants, opinion surveys, and historical overviews may be helpful in identifying these influencing factors.

The value of any resource analysis is dependent upon the thoroughness of the investigation. There may be duplication of services, lack of coordination, and little communication among agencies or individuals involved in the provision of care. There may even be rivalry or territoriality between health care providers, which may limit or influence the interpretation of information. A relatively large community may produce an overwhelming amount of information requiring a great deal of time spent on classification and explanation. A very small community may rely on individual health care users as their informants.

Seldom is one community a self-contained unit that can provide for the total needs of its members. Therefore, a comprehensive resource analysis often requires a survey of the availability of resources in the larger society.

The definition of community assessment, its purposes, and factors affecting its focus have been discussed. A number of techniques used in performing a community assessment are described. Each technique provides different information. It is often necessary to use a combination of techniques in order to obtain the information a nurse needs to provide health care to a community.

REFERENCES

1. BLUM, H: *Planning for Health.* Human Sciences Press, New York, 1974.

2. BECKER, M (ED): *The Health Belief Model and Personal Health Behavior.* Charles B. Slack, Thorofare, NJ, 1974, p 22.

3. US DEPARTMENT OF HEALTH, EDUCATION, AND WELFARE: *Vital Statistics of the United States.* National Center for Health Statistics, Division of Vital Statistics (Published annually), Hyattsville, MD.

4. CENTER FOR DISEASE CONTROL: *Morbidity and Mortality Weekly Report,* Atlanta.

5. US SUPERINTENDENT OF DOCUMENTS: *Vital and Health Statistics* (Published annually), Washington, DC.

6. BUREAU OF CENSUS, US DEPARTMENT OF COMMERCE: *1980 Census of Population and Housing.* Bureau of Census, US Department of Commerce, Washington, DC, 1983.

7. BABBIE, E: *Survey Research Methods.* Wadsworth, Belmont, CA, 1973.

8. Ibid.

UNIT BIBLIOGRAPHY

ARCHER, SE AND FLESHMAN, RP: *Community Health Nursing: Patterns and Practice,* ed 2. Duxbury Press, North Scituate, MA, 1979.

BABBIE, E: *Survey Research Methods.* Wadsworth, Belmont, CA, 1973.

BECKER, M (ED): *The Health Belief Model and Personal Health Behavior.* Charles B. Slack, Thorofare, NJ, 1974, p 22.

BLUM, H: *Planning for Health.* Human Sciences, New York, 1974.

BRADEN, CJ AND HERBAN, NL: *Community Health: A Systems Approach.* Appleton-Century-Crofts, New York, 1976.

BROWNLEE, AT: *Community, Culture, and Care: A Cross-Cultural Guide for Health Workers.* CV Mosby, St Louis, 1978.

BUREAU OF CENSUS, US DEPARTMENT OF COMMERCE: *1980 Census of Population and Housing.* Bureau of Census, US Department of Commerce, Washington, DC, 1983.

BURGESS, W AND ROGLAND, EC: *Community Health Nursing: Philosophy, Process, Practice.* Appleton-Century-Crofts, Norwalk, CN, 1983.

CENTER FOR DISEASE CONTROL: *Morbidity and Mortality Weekly Report* (Published weekly), Atlanta.

CLEMEN, SA, EIGSTI, DG, MCGUIRE, SL: *Comprehensive Family and Community Health Nursing.* McGraw-Hill, New York, 1981.

CONNOR, DM: *Understanding Your Community*, ed 2. Development Press, Ottawa, Canada, 1969.

CORDES, S: *Assessing health care needs: Elements and process.* Family and Community Health, Vol 1 (2), August 1978, pp 1–16.

COX, F, ET AL: *Tactics and Techniques of Community Practice.* FE Peacock Publications, Itasca, IL, 1977.

DEVER, A: *Community Health Analysis: A Holistic Approach.* Aspen, Germantown, MD, 1980.

ELINSON, J AND SIEGMANN A (EDS): *Sociomedical Health Indicators.* Boywood, Farmingdale, NY, 1979.

EXECUTIVE COMMITTEE AND THE STANDARDS COMMITTEE OF THE AMERICAN NURSES ASSOCIATION: *Standards of Nursing Practice.* American Nurses Association, Kansas City, MO, 1973.

FABER, M AND REINHARDT, A: *Promoting Health Through Risk Reduction.* Macmillan, New York, 1982.

FREEMAN, R AND HEINRICH, J: *Community Health Nursing Practice.* WB Saunders, Philadelphia, 1981.

FROMER, M: *Community Health Care and the Nursing Process.* CV Mosby, St Louis, 1979.

HALL, J AND WEAVER B: *Distributive Nursing Practice: A Systems Approach to Community Health.* JB Lippincott, Philadelphia, 1977.

HANLON, J AND PICKETT, G: *Public Health Administration and Practice.* CV Mosby, St Louis, 1979.

HELVIE, C: *Community Health Nursing Theory and Process.* Harper & Row, New York, 1981.

HILLEBOE, H AND LARIMORE, G: *Preventive Medicine.* WB Saunders, Philadelphia, 1966.

JARVIS, L: *Community Health Nursing: Keeping the Public Healthy.* FA Davis, Philadelphia, 1981.

KURTZMAN, C, ET AL: *Nursing process at the aggregate level.* Nurs Outlook, December 1980, pp 737–739.

LEAHY, K, COBB, M, JONES, M: *Community Health Nursing,* ed 4. McGraw-Hill, New York, 1982.

MASLOW, AH: *Motivation and Personality,* ed 2. Harper & Row, New York, 1970.

SACKET, D, ET AL: *The development and application of indices of health: General methods and a summary of results.* Am J Public Health 67:423, May 1977.

SHAMANSKY, S AND PEZNECKER, B: *A community is. . . .* In SPRADLEY, BW (ED): *Readings in Community Health Nursing.* Boston, Little, Brown & Co, 1982 (originally published in Nursing Outlook, Vol 29, No 3, 1981).

SPRADLEY, BW: *Community Health Nursing Concepts and Practice.* Little, Brown & Co, Boston, 1981.

STEWART, R: *Human Services Needs Assessment.* Ph.D. Dissertation, California School of Professional Psychology, Fresno, CA, 1978 (University Microfilms International, Ann Arbor, MI).

STEWART, R: *The nature of needs assessment in community mental health.* Community Ment Health J 15(4):287, 1979.

STEWART, R AND POASTER, L: *Methods of assessing mental and physical health needs from social statistics. Evaluation* 2:67, 1975.

TINKHAM, C AND VOORHIES, E: *Community Health Nursing: Evolution and Process.* Appleton-Century-Crofts, New York, 1972.

US DEPARTMENT OF HEALTH, EDUCATION AND WELFARE: *Healthy People.* The Surgeon General's Report on Health Promotion and Disease Prevention. PHS Publication #79-550717, Washington, DC, 1979.

US DEPARTMENT OF HEALTH, EDUCATION, AND WELFARE: *Vital Statistics of the United States.* National Center for Health Statistics, Division of Vital Statistics (Published annually), Hyattsville, MD.

US SUPERINTENDENT OF DOCUMENTS: *Vital and Health Statistics (Published annually),* Washington, DC.

WARHEIT, G, BELL, R, SCHWAS, J: *Needs Assessment Approaches: Concepts and Methods.* US Department of Health, Education and Welfare, Washington, DC, 1979.

WARREN, RL: *The Community in America,* ed 2. Rand McNally, New York, 1973.

WARREN, RL (ED): *Perspective on the American Community.* Rand McNally, Chicago, 1966.

WILLIAMS, C: *Community health nursing—what is it?:* In SPRADLEY, BW (ED): *Readings in Community Health Nursing.* ed 2. Boston, Little, Brown & Co, 1982 (previously published in Nursing Outlook Vol 25, No 4, pp 250–254).

CONCEPTUAL APPROACHES TO COMMUNITY ASSESSMENT

There are a number of conceptual approaches which might be used in performing a community assessment. This unit describes selected approaches drawn from nursing and other disciplines. Each approach includes both content and process. The content is concerned with what is contained within the limits described for that community, such as its structure and functions. The process describes the relationships that occur among the various elements within the community and its environment. The emphasis on content or process varies with the approach. The assessment must be based upon an approach that is appropriate for the situation, the philosophy and abilities of the investigative participants, and the audience for which the results are intended.

CHAPTER 3

EPIDEMIOLOGICAL APPROACH TO COMMUNITY ASSESSMENT

OBJECTIVES

THE LEARNER WILL

1. define common terms related to epidemiology and biostatistics.

2. differentiate between an incidence rate and a prevalence rate.

3. interpret census tract data in a community assessment.

4. use results of epidemiological research to determine "at risk" status of a population.

5. apply the steps of an epidemiological investigation in exploring an increased incidence of a health disorder.

Epidemiology is a foundational science in community health. It is one of the most commonly used approaches to study and to describe the health status of a community. Nurses constantly use information obtained from epidemiological research to provide health counseling and direct service to individual clients and families. For instance, the relationships between life style habits and development of many forms of cardiopulmonary diseases and cancer have been determined through epidemiological research. This information is the basis for much of the health counseling provided by nurses. Nurses may be called upon to participate in epidemiological investigations and to interpret their results to the community.

WHAT IS EPIDEMIOLOGY?

Although the epidemiological approach has been used since ancient times, modern epidemiology is dated from the beginning of the 20th century prior to the acceptance of the germ theory. The term epidemiology referred to a medical science that investigated epidemics "with the objective of tracing their sources, limiting their spread and introducing measures to control existing epidemics and preventing future occurrences."[1] Epidemic refers to an unusually high occurrence of disease in a population and classically refers to communicable or infectious diseases. Leavell and Clark define epidemiology as "a field of science which is concerned with the various factors and conditions that determine the occurrence and distribution of health, disease, defect, disability and death among groups of individuals."[2] Furthermore, Paul indicates in Leavell and Clark that epidemiology is "concerned with the circumstances under which disease occurs, where diseases tend to flourish and where they do not. Such circumstances may be microbiological or toxicological, they may be based on genetic, social or environmental factors, even religious or political factors may come under scrutiny provided they are found to have some bearing upon disease prevalence."[3] Each condition has its pattern of progression or "natural history." An understanding of this pattern assists in determining points of intervention.[4]

Although there are a number of examples of the use of the epidemiological approach to study noninfectious disease—particularly focusing upon occupational hazards—the 1950s demonstrated a great surge in use of this approach to study the health problems that plague developed industrialized nations, for example, cancer, heart disease, hypertension, accidents, mental and social disorders. With this broadening of focus came a broadening of definition. Susser provides a definition much more in keeping with the current usage of the term, one which is more useful to nursing practice and community assessment.

Epidemiology is the study of the distribution and determinants of *states of health* in human populations . . . these activities are for the purpose of the prevention, surveillance, and control of *health disorders* in populations. Therefore, epidemiology fosters the practice of preventive care. As knowledge of factors and characteristics which cause, predict or are associated with the development of health disorders become uncovered, individuals who are at high risk for developing the health disorder can be identified and preventive measures undertaken.[5]

Therefore, as society changed and the infectious diseases were conquered with the use of immunizations, antibiotics, and improved sanitary conditions, the focus of epidemiological investigations shifted to the study of chronic diseases. This occurred around the middle of the 20th century. A comprehensive description of such studies may be found in Litienfield and Gifford's[6] book, *Chronic Disease and Public Health*.

Regardless of definition, epidemiology is a process that 1) is based on scientific inquiry, 2) recognizes the involvement of many influencing factors, 3) has as its laboratory the community, and 4) is concerned with a population or group of people. In order to select and to interpret data necessary to describe the occurrence and distribution of health disorders, multiple interactive factors must be considered. Leavell and Clark[7] suggest that knowledge of the following factors is essential: 1) clinical medicine for the clinical history, assessment, and diagnosis of the health disorder (or clinical nursing when investigating nursing diagnoses); 2) microbiology for knowledge of living agents of disease; 3) chemistry and physical sciences, particularly for recognition of health hazards in the environment; 4) demography—composition and characteristics of populations; 5) anthropology and sociology for cultural and sociological characteristics of populations; 6) genetics and psychology for personal characteristics which may influence health disorders; 7) meteorology and topography for weather, climate, and structure of land masses; and 8) biostatistics—the basic tools for data collection and analysis, including vital statistics—regarding natality, mortality, and morbidity. Thus, use of an epidemiological approach to assess a community requires knowledge of a number of key concepts.

FRAMEWORKS USEFUL TO EPIDEMIOLOGY

Host-Agent-Environment Triad

Classically the conceptual model used to organize and to analyze interactive factors in disease occurrence was the Host-Agent-Environment Triad (H-A-E Triad) depicted in Figure 3-1.

Epidemiological investigators are concerned with identifying the who, what, and where in the development of disorders. The host in the triad is the "who" in epidemiology: those persons susceptible to developing the health disorder. The "what" refers to the agent or factors that cause or are associated with the health disorder. The environment is the "where," or all the external conditions within which the interaction of the agent and host takes place. Any change in one of the three aspects of the triad affects the balance of the factors influencing health, thereby increasing or decreasing the risk of development of a health

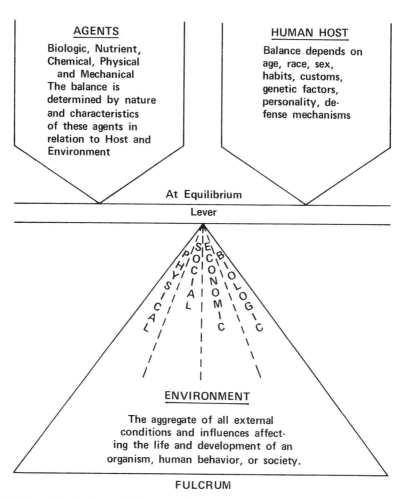

FIGURE 3-1. Illustration of factors influencing health equilibrium modified from Leavell and Clark.[1]

disorder in the human host. For instance, a change in the host's ability to resist infection, a new strain of influenza virus for which antibodies have not been developed, or a change in climate or weather pattern will all affect an individual's chances of developing the flu.

Reciprocal Systems Model

As the study of health disorders demonstrated multiple causation and clarified the interrelationships among these factors, certain limitations in the H-A-E Triad model were noted. Often the agent(s) or cause(s) were intrinsic to the definition of the host itself or of the environment. Therefore a model with reciprocal inter-

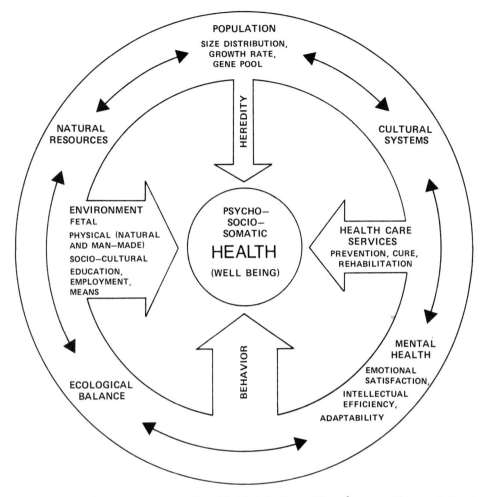

FIGURE 3-2. The Environment of Health Model. (From Blum,[9] p. 3, with permission.)

active parts was developed to depict factors affecting health. Figure 3-2 is an example of such a model.

In his forward to the book *Healthy People*, Joseph Califano, the secretary of HEW in 1979, remarks upon the interactive nature of factors affecting health and the results of the tremendous effort in epidemiological research over the last few decades. He states,

> I can compress what we have learned about the causes of modern killers in three summarizing sentences.
> We are killing ourselves by our own careless habits.
> We are killing ourselves by carelessly polluting the environment.
> We are killing ourselves by permitting harmful social conditions to

persist—conditions like poverty, hunger and ignorance which destroy health, especially for infants and children.[8]

Holistic Model

At the same time the reciprocal interactive models were being developed, the concept of holism, or the holistic health approach, evolved in the nursing and health-related literature. According to Blum, "Holistic means . . . viewing a person and his/her wellness from every possible perspective. . . . It means treating the person not the disease. The holistic approach promotes an interrelationship and unity of body, mind and spirit."[9]

Health versus Illness Model

Along with this holistic approach, the development of a focus on health rather than on illness has occurred. This shift in focus has become very popular. It is a current trend in health and nursing literature. This has had an impact on epidemiological research. Susser states that the World Health Organization definition of health ("complete physical, mental and social well-being and not just the absence of disease") has not been made operational. Rather, he says, "We tend to describe and measure health as the obverse of disease, illness and sickness or of impairment, disability and handicap. . . . In this epidemiology describes the occurrence and evolution of these disordered states of health and seeks to discover their causes and prevent them."[10] Dever[11] notes that death certificates code diseases, *not* true *cause* of death. He suggests that instead of listing heart attack, lung cancer, and so forth as the cause of death on the death certificate, such things as lack of exercise, inadequate diet, smoking, excessive drinking, and air pollution should be listed. One would then have the 10 leading causes of death rather than the top 10 diseases with which people died. Interestingly, sociomedical health indices are being developed to provide alternative definitions of the health of populations.

STATISTICS—THE LANGUAGE OF EPIDEMIOLOGY

Biostatistics refers to "the science which deals with the plans and methods of collecting, tabulating, and analyzing numerical facts and figures in the life sciences."[12] A basic understanding of biostatistics is important for the nurse to interpret epidemiological research findings and to organize data for a community assessment.

In the introduction to the epidemiological approach, the term *epidemic* was used to refer to the occurrence of health disorders in a defined population which was in excess of the usual or normally expected number of cases in that population. The term *endemic* is used to refer to the amount of a health disorder that is usually or normally occurring in that defined population. If a disease is said to be endemic in a particular locale, it means that condition is commonly found there. Therefore, in order to determine if there is an epidemic, there has to be a sense of what is "normal" for that community. There must be some form of measurement to determine the amounts of a specific health disorder in a defined population and to describe its distribution among subgroups within that population. This form of measurement must go beyond that of a count in order to provide for comparisons—over time, among subgroups, between that population and other populations, or against some external standard. It is through these comparisons that the nurse can determine whether the community's (client's) health status is getting "better" or "worse" and if members of that community are at particular risk for the development of certain health disorders. Therefore, an understanding of common statistics used in describing health behavior in populations will help the nurse interpret published data and to determine the kind of data needed in order to assess the community or an outbreak of a health disorder.

When counting occurrences of a health disorder in a community, the first statistic formulated is usually a *frequency distribution*. For example, three cases of measles were reported to the health department on May 1, seven cases on May 2, ten cases on May 3, and so on. This may be summarized with some indication of the *proportion* of the total number of incidents or responses. If there were 100 incidents of measles reported in May, then 3% were reported on May 1, 7% on May 2, 10% on May 3, and so on (Fig. 3-3). In this way, the pattern of occurrence of an episode or outbreak of a health disorder is determined.

This technique forms the basis for descriptive statistics used in studying a community. The characteristics of a population described in the data published

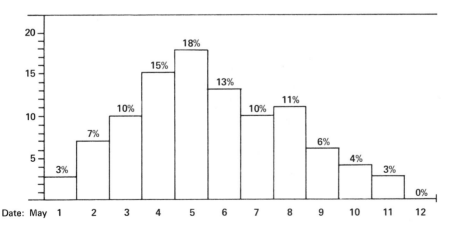

FIGURE 3-3. Distribution of cases of measles, May 1984.

by the Bureau of Census provide a picture of the community in terms of the distribution of the population by age categories, race, sex, and socioeconomic indicators. These figures can be used to easily determine, for instance, the proportion of elderly residing in a given area.

Another statistic which may be included in such data describes what is called the *central tendency* of responses or count within the distribution of responses. Most familiar are the arithmetic mean (the average) and the median (or the value which lies in the middle of the distribution of a set of numbers). These statistical measures can be used to describe the characteristics of a population and even to compare neighborhoods within a community with each other or with the community as a whole.

As an example, Table 3-1 provides a comparison of two very different geographic areas within Spokane, Washington. Geographic areas can be divided into smaller areas known as census tracts for the purpose of counting and describing the population therein. In this illustration, census tract number 34 is adjacent to the downtown commercial area and is what might be referred to as the "skid row" area. Census tract 128 is in the "Valley," or suburb of Spokane. An analysis of this data leads the nurse to draw the following conclusions, identify potential health needs, and priorities in services:

> The population in census tract 34 is primarily older unemployed, single individuals having less than a high school diploma, living on marginal incomes in one-room rental apartments in older multiple dwelling units which often lack kitchen facilities and share bathroom facilities, paying minimal rent and not owning a car. In comparison, the population in census tract 128 is primarily young married couples with about two school-age children. The parents are high school graduates or have attended college; their income is higher than the city average, and a large portion of the families have both parents working in professional or "white collar" jobs. These families own single dwelling units built within the last 10 years which have about six rooms and are valued at about twice that of the overall city median. These families own at least one and usually more cars.

Additional statistical procedures to assure comparability are required to make comparisons among groups of people regarding their health status. To indicate there are 10 cases of measles is meaningless unless you know whether those 10 cases occurred in a classroom of 25 second graders or in a city of 250,000 people. Therefore, statistical procedures called rates and ratios are formulated. A *rate* is the total number of occurrences of a condition divided by the total population at risk of developing that condition.

$$\text{Rate} = \frac{\text{Number of persons affected}}{\text{Total population at risk of being affected}} \times \text{Constant}$$

The numerator is always a proportion of those in the denominator. This is often a small number. For instance, a measles case rate of 0.004 second graders is difficult—both to conceptualize because people are not divisible and to discuss in comparison with a rate in a different population. Therefore, the rate or number is usually multiplied by a "constant," for example, 1,000 or 100,000. The rate is then reported as four cases of measles per 1000 second graders.

There are a number of rates that are used to describe the health status of a population. *Morbidity rates* describe the amount of disease occurring in a population. Vital statistics, which are drawn from certificates filed with the county government, include data related to natality (from birth certificates), mortality (from death certificates), and marriages and dissolutions of marriage (from corresponding certificates). Formulas for calculation of rates based on these data are easily obtainable from biostatistic books.

In reviewing or constructing morbidity statistics it is important to differentiate between incidence and prevalence. These two words are often confused in the public media. The *incidence rate* refers to the number of *new* cases in a population during a given time period and describes the *development* of a health disorder in a community. The *prevalence rate* refers to the *total* number of cases of a health disorder in a population at a particular time regardless of whether the cases are *new or old*.

$$\text{Incidence Rate} = \frac{\text{Number of new cases of a health disorder}}{\text{Population at risk during a given time period}} \times \text{Constant}$$

$$\text{Prevalence Rate} = \frac{\text{Total number of cases of a health disorder}}{\text{Population at risk at a date or point in time}} \times \text{Constant}$$

The incidence of tuberculosis (TB) in a community would be the number of new cases reported during a period of time in that community; the prevalence of TB would be the total number of TB cases existing in that community at that time. One might have an incidence rate of 1 per 100,000 people and a prevalence of 5 per 100,000 people for January 1, 1982.

Because the incidence rate measures the rate of new cases occurring in a population, it indicates the need for preventive measures, assists in evaluating current control measures, and provides direction for program planning. It may be used for both acute and chronic conditions. However, because of the length of time many chronic conditions take to develop prior to diagnosis, it is less useful in directing immediate preventive measures with these conditions.

A prevalence rate measures the magnitude of a health disorder in a given population at a given time. It indicates the need for services, economic loss to the community, and provides direction for program planning and evaluation. The prevalence rate is commonly used with chronic conditions or those conditions with a duration of months or years.

In interpreting incidence and prevalence rates, the nurse must consider factors that may affect these rates. Both rates may increase or decrease owing to a shift in population characteristics. If a new urban development greatly increases the number of young families in a community, the incidence of childhood dis-

TABLE 3-1. Comparison Among Spokane City and Select Census Tracts on Certain 1970 Census Data*

	CITY OF SPOKANE	34 LOW†	128 HIGH†
Population	170,516	1,638	4,228
Black	2,161 (1.3%)	40 (2.4%)	—
Age: <5 (5 yr span)	13,005 (7.6%)	6 (0.4%)	367 (8.7%)
5-19 (15 yr span)	46,884 (27.5%)	34 (2.1%)	1,647 (40%)
20-44 (25 yr span)	48,276 (28.3%)	200 (12.2%)	1,387 (32.8%)
45-59 (15 yr span)	29,841 (17.5%)	427 (26.1%)	668 (15.8%)
>60 (15 + yr span)	32,510 (19 %)	971 (59.3%)	159 (3.8%)
% Males/%Females	M = 47.4% F = 52.6%	M = 80% F = 20%	M = 49.8% F = 50.2%
Marital Status (14 + older)	130,417	1,629	2,813
Single	31,592 (24.2%)	663 (40.7%)	703 (25%)
Married	78,425 (60.1%)	264 (16.2%)	2,014 (71.6%)
Separated	1,966 (1.5%)	93 (5.7%)	12 (0.4%)
Widowed	12,800 (9.8%)	271 (16.6%)	55 (1.9%)
Divorced	7,600 (5.8%)	431 (26.5%)	41 (1.5%)
% Ages 16-21 Not in school, not high school graduates (dropouts)	(7.9%)	(25.0%)	—
Highest education of persons ≥25 in %			
8 yrs or less	(19.3%)	(58.4%)	(4.2%)
9-12 yrs	(62.1%)	(35 %)	(47.3%)
1 or more yrs of college	(27.4%)	(6 %)	(47.6%)
Median school years	12.4	8.8	13
% High school graduates	64%	22.2%	88%
Income: Number of families	43,516	98‡	1,025
Median	$ 9,137	$ 2,840	$13,785
Mean	$10,295	$ 5,788	$14,780
% Receiving Social Security	23.3%	46.9%	6.6%
% Receiving public assistance	6 %	39.8%	0.9%
% Below poverty level	9.3%	39.8%	1.1%

Employment Status			
Men ≥16 yrs, % in labor force	61,873 (70.6%)	(24.7%)	(87.8%)
Women ≥ 16 yrs, % in labor force	(40.11%)	(32.1%)	(40.5%)
Occupation: Total			
Employed ≥16 yrs	(35.1%)	333 (18%)	1,537 (52%)
Professional, technical, administrative, and sales			
Year-round housing—Total	64,321	1,619	1,171
Units in structure: 1	48,948 [76 %]	1,594 (98.4%)	1,117 (95.3%)
5 or more	10,215 [15 %]	15 (0.9%)	—
Year Built: 1960-1970	5,997 [92 %]	12 (0.7%)	836 (71.3%)
Before 1939	34,492 [53 %]	1,102 (98.9%)	6 (0.5%)
Heating Equipment: Steam	9,989 [15 %]	1,454 (89.8%)	115 (9.82%)
Warm air	41,545 [64 %]	96 (5.9%)	980 (83.6%)
Equipment: More than 1 bath	14,599 [22 %]	—	989 (84.4%)
Units lacking some or all plumbing	3,037 [4.7%]	1,188 (75 %)	3 (0.3%)
Units lacking complete kitchen facilities	1,928 [3 %]	483 (30.5%)	32 (2.7%)
Median rooms	4.8	1.3	6.6
Cars: None	11,419 [17 %]	1,110 (86.5%)	—
2 or more	21,085 [32 %]	7 (0.5%)	886 (75.5%)
Structure: Owner occupied	40,134 [62.4%]	9 (0.5%)	999 (85.3%)
All occupied housing units	60,512	1,283	1,066
Median persons—owner occupied	2.5	1.4	4.0
Median persons—renter occupied	1.7	1.0	3.5
Median value—in $	$12,500	—	$25,900
Median contract rent—in $	71	45	163

*Data drawn from Higgs, Z: 1970 Census of Population and Housing, Census Tracts for Spokane, Washington Standard Metropolitan Statistical Area. Bureau of Census, Washington, DC, 1972.

†Designations of high, medium, and low are based on composite scores, using three factors—median income, percent high school graduates, and percent skilled/unskilled labor, as determined by the Spokane County Health District.

‡By family; not individual and tract 34 very low proportion of families.

eases during the years the community is in transition may rise. However, if that housing development is for senior citizens, then the prevalence of certain chronic conditions will rise. Development of new technology, such as vaccine, may sharply drop the incidence rate. However, advances in technology that save lives but do not cure the disease raise the prevalence rate. Diabetes is one example of this phenomenon. Increased interest, services, and funds poured into coping with a health condition may mean better and earlier diagnosis, an increased awareness, and, therefore, better reporting of that health disorder. This raises the incidence rate. Therefore, an investigation of factors causing a shift in these rates must be accomplished before program planning is instituted.

An *attack rate* is a morbidity rate that is often used to describe the portion of people exposed to a disease who develop the disease. This is extremely important in an epidemiological investigation. Particularly with food poisonings, an attack rate is calculated for both individuals who become ill and those who did not for each food eaten or not eaten. This helps identify which foods are suspect for carrying organisms or toxins. An attack rate also is a measure of the severity of the problem. If five people are exposed to a health hazard and all five develop the disease, the attack rate is 100%. If one of the five develops the disease, the attack rate is 20%.

There are two basic kinds of death rates or *mortality rates:* a crude death rate and a rate that is specific according to some characteristic. The crude death rate refers to all persons dying of all causes in a given population during a given time. Examples of specific rates would be age specific (for example, infant mortality rate), disease or cause specific (for example, by diagnosis—diabetes, influenza), or a combination of the two (for example, the rate of deaths of children under the age of 1 from accidents in the state of Washington in 1982.) Rates may be calculated for any size population from local to international. Table 3-2, taken from World Health Organization data, uses some of the previously identified statistical measures to make rough comparisons of the health status of various nations. For instance, during 1977 about one child out of 100, or 1.4% of the children, born in the United States died before 1 year of age. In Afghanistan, about 22 children in 100, 22.6% or about 1 in 4, of the children born there die before 1 year of age.

Table 3-2 provides a "rough" comparison among groups. There is a statistical procedure commonly used in biostatistics which more specifically compares the rate of one group with that of another. This is called a *ratio* and is created by dividing one rate by another. For instance, if the lung cancer death rate for smokers is 188 per 100,000 and the lung cancer death rate for nonsmokers is 19 per 100,000, then the ratio is 9.9 to 1. This is often reported as 9.9 times greater risk.[13]

$$\frac{\text{Smoker lung cancer rate: } 188/100,000}{\text{Nonsmoker lung cancer rate: } 19/100,000} = \text{Ratio of } 9.9{:}1$$

Other examples from the Surgeon General's Report—*Healthy People* comparing race and sex include the facts that blacks between the ages of 15 and

TABLE 3-2. World Health Statistic

COUNTRY	BIRTH RATE	DEATH RATE	INFANT MORTALITY	% POP < 15	% POP > 64	LIFE EXPECT-ANCY	POLI*	GNP (US)†
Sweden	12	11	8	21	15	75	97	9,250
Japan	15	6	9	24	8	75	96	5,640
France	14	10	11	24	14	73	95	7,290
E Germany	13	13	13	21	16	72	94	4,940
United Kingdom	12	12	14	23	14	72	94	4,430
Canada	16	7	14	26	8	76	95	8,450
US‡	15	9	14	24	11	73	95	8,640
Puerto Rico	23	6	18	35	7	72	90	2,460
Israel	20	7	20	33	8	73	89	2,920
USSR	18	10	30	26	9	70	91	3,010
China	20	8	56	35	5	64	71	410
Mexico	41	7	70	46	3	65	75	1,110
Iran	44	14	104	45	3	57	52	2,180
Egypt	38	12	108	41	3	55	44	310
India	34	15	122	41	3	50	41	150
United Arab Emirates	44	14	138	34	3	48	34	14,420
Algeria	48	14	142	48	4	54	41	1,110
Swaziland	47	19	168	48	3	44	33	580
Afghanistan	50	27	226	44	3	39	17	190

Rates per 1000 population. Data refer to 1976 or 1977 statistics and are drawn from Population Reference Bureau: *1979 World Population Data Sheet.* Washington, DC.

*POLI: Physical Life Index (combines infant mortality, life expectancy, and literacy, with low = 0; high = 100).

†Per capita Gross National Product.

‡20 countries have an equal or lower infant mortality and 144 have a higher infant mortality than the US.

24 are five times as likely to be murdered as whites of the same age, and traumatic deaths in men between the ages of 15 and 24 are close to four times that of women in the same age group.[14] Another ratio commonly used is the proportion of persons having a disease who died of that disease during a given year. This is a *case-fatality* ratio and gives an estimate of the probability of dying from a disease.

Another use of ratio is to compare a group(s) with an outside standard. For instance, in studying the effects of smoking on lung cancer, the outside standard might be the death rate of lung cancer in nonsmokers. Various categories of smokers based on amount and length of smoking would be compared with those who do not smoke to determine differences in risk. A second example of the use of a standard is the concept of endemic incidence in a population. There is usually a level at which a condition is considered endemic. An expected incidence of a disease based on the history of the development of the disease in that population becomes a standard against which a certain episode of a disease is judged epidemic. A third standard is the disease rate in a population. It can be used to compare the rates of subgroups within the population which differ on some factor. For instance, comparing the suicide rates of various age groups within a population with the overall suicide rate identifies high-risk age groups. This approach identifies factors associated with a condition that deserve further investigation.

For instance, Friedman[15] reports a study by Kagen and Kennel to determine the relationship between blood pressure and coronary heart disease. They found that individuals with systolic blood pressure (BP) of 120 mm Hg or below had an incidence rate that was only 33 percent the expected incidence of coronary heart disease in the overall population, whereas those individuals whose systolic BP was at least 180 mm Hg experienced 223 percent the expected incidence. The expected incidence was based on the experience of the total population studied and was used as the standard for comparison.

CONCEPT OF "AT RISK"

Another concept that is referred to frequently in the epidemiology and health literature is the concept of being "at risk." This concept has particular relevance for nursing and community assessment.

The population at risk refers to those persons susceptible to a health disorder and is used as the denominator in calculating rates. For instance, in determining the rate of cancer of the cervix in a particular community, the population at risk would not be the total population in the community but only the female population. Determining exactly who is to be included in this population at risk is sometimes difficult, and in these instances the rates constructed are limited in their accuracy.

The same concept is used when referring to a "high-risk population." High-risk population is used to denote a specific classification of people for whom research has determined particularly high rates of a health disorder. This concept is focused on the "who" in epidemiology, or the susceptible host, and in an epidemiological investigation is often classified by age, sex, ethnicity, and socioeconomic status; for example, income, education, marital status, religion, life style characteristics. For instance, studies indicate that "an American man, compared to a Japanese man of the same age is at 1.5 times higher risk of death from all causes, 5 times higher for death from heart disease and 4 times higher for death from lung cancer. And for breast cancer, the death rate for American women is four times as great as the Japanese woman. On the other hand, a Japanese man is eight times as likely to die from stomach cancer than his American counterpart."[16] Figure 3-4 demonstrates differences in the infant mortality rates by race in the U.S.

As noted in *Healthy People*, "yet, despite the progress [in reduction of infant mortality], the first year of life remains the most hazardous period until age 65, and black infants are nearly twice as likely to die before their first birthdays as white infants. The death rate in 1977 for black infants is about the same as that for white infants 25 years ago."[17] Table 3-3 provides data regarding conditions for which each age group is at high risk.

An important principle related to the concept of high-risk populations is the synergistic effect of factors in the production of health disorders—"the com-

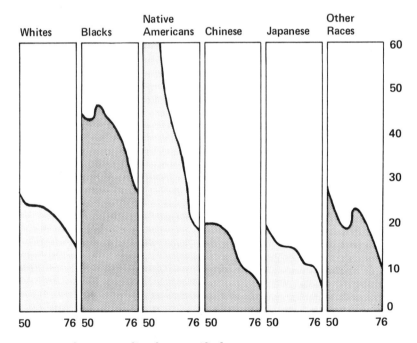

FIGURE 3-4. Infant mortality by specified race, 1950–1976. 1976 rates: 15.2 (all groups). Rates per 1000 live births. (From US Department of Health, Education and Welfare: *Health Status of Minorities and Low-Income Groups.* HRA Publication #79-627. Washington, DC, p 38.)

TABLE 3-3. Causes of Death by Life Stages, 1977

PROBLEM / AGE GROUPS	INFANTS (UNDER 1) RANK	RATE*	CHILDREN (1-14) RANK	RATE†	ADOLESCENTS/YOUNG ADULTS (15-24) RANK	RATE†	ADULTS (25-44) RANK	RATE†	ADULTS (45-64) RANK	RATE†	OLDER ADULTS (OVER 65) RANK	RATE†	TOTAL POPULATION (ALL AGES) RANK	RATE†
Chronic Diseases														
Heart Disease			7	1.1	6	2.5	2	25.5	1	351.0	1	2334.1	1	332.3
Stroke			8	.6	9	1.2	8	6.1	3	52.4	3	658.2	3	84.1
Arteriosclerosis											5	116.5	9	13.3
Bronchitis, Emphysema, & Asthma									10	12.2	8	69.3		
Cancer			3	4.9	5	6.5	1	29.7	2	302.7	2	988.5	2	178.7
Diabetes Mellitus					10	.4	10	2.4	8	17.8	6	100.5	7	15.2
Cirrhosis of the Liver							7	8.6	4	39.2	9	36.7	8	14.3
Infectious Diseases														
Influenza and Pneumonia	5	50.6	6	1.5	8	1.3	9	3.0	9	15.3	4	169.7	5	23.7
Meningitis			8	.6										
Septicemia	6	32.7												
Trauma														
Accidents														
Motor vehicle accidents			2	9.0	1	44.1	3	23.1	7	18.3	10	24.5	6	22.9
All other accidents	7	27.7	1	10.8	2	18.4	4	18.5	5	25.5	7	78.1	4	24.8
Suicide			10	.4	3	13.6	5	17.3	6	19.1			9	13.3
Homicide			5	1.6	4	12.7	6	15.6						
Developmental Problems														
Immaturity associated	1	407.7												
Birth-associated	2	294.4												
Congenital birth defects	3	253.1	4	3.6	7	1.6								
Sudden infant deaths	4	142.8												
All causes		1412.1		43.1		117.1		182.5		1,000.0		5288.1		878.1

*Rate per 100,000 live births.
†Rate per 100,000 population in specified group.
Source: Based on data from the National Center for Health Statistics, Division of Vital Statistics.

bined potential for harm of many risk factors is more than the sum of their individual effects."[18] For example, research has determined that asbestos workers have increased lung cancer risk. "Asbestos workers who smoke have 30 times more risk than coworkers who do not smoke and 90 times more than people who neither smoke nor work with asbestos." The report concludes, "It is the controllability of many risks and, often, the significance of controlling even only a few that lies at the heart of disease prevention and health promotion."[19]

From such studies researchers have determined factors that are statistically related to or associated with health disorders. According to Dever, "Association refers to the relationship that may exist between the occurrence of one thing and the occurrence of another, e.g., between a risk factor and a health disorder."[20] Frequently in both medical and nursing literature, a discussion of a particular health disorder is introduced by an explanation of its etiology or the complex of causative factors, including contributing or predisposing factors that have been found to be related to the condition. It is beyond the scope of this chapter to discuss the stringent criteria required by epidemiological research to determine that an association is causal. But much of the basis for health counseling comes from the knowledge of these associations and resultant identification of high-risk populations.*

MECHANISM OF TRANSMISSION

Closely related to this concept of populations at risk is a model originally developed to describe the mechanism of transmission of infectious organisms[21] but which with some "stretching" can be used to describe the chain of events in the epidemiology of any health disorder. Table 3-4 depicts the use of this model with noninfectious health disorders at a fairly simplistic level. As indicated in this table, the points of intervention may be determined along the chain of events in the development of a health disorder. Reduction of irritants in industrial exhaust would intervene at the avenue of escape level, whereas use of a mask for workers in highly dusty areas would intervene at the portal of entry level. One major limitation of the model is that it does not account for the interaction of multiple factors but describes the relationship of each factor to the health disorder.

EPIDEMIOLOGICAL RESEARCH

Epidemiological studies use a wide range of research approaches. Some studies are *descriptive* in nature. Their intent is to describe the situation clearly. Once a

---

*For an excellent description of criteria used to judge that an association is causal, refer to Susser, M: *Causal Thinking in Health Sciences.* Oxford University Press, New York, 1975, p 140.

TABLE 3-4. Health Disorder from an Epidemiological Viewpoint

CONDITION	AGENT (Causal or associated factor)	AVENUE OF ESCAPE (Path by which agent leaves normal habitat)	MODE OF CONVEYANCE (Essential mechanism to bridge gap between agent's exit and source of entry of susceptible host)	PORTAL OF ENTRY (Site at which agent interacts with host)	HOST (Especially high-risk population)
Chronic bronchitis	Chemical/ mechanical irritant	Smoke, exhaust	Air	Inhaled into lungs irritates bronchial mucosal lining	Males, smokers, urban-dwellers, occupations with high dust or fumes
Arteriosclerotic heart disease	Chronic psychological stress, aging(?), high cholesterol, high saturated fats, hypertension, obesity, low levels of exercise	Industrialized life style; Contained in animal food; sedentary habits	Ingestion, absorbed through GI tract, builds in vascular walls, arteriosclerosis	Technologically advanced societies, males, smokers, familial history of high levels of cholesterol and lipids in blood	

clear description of the phenomenon or situation is available, an *analytical* approach is used to determine relationships among factors. The studies determining different degrees of risk of developing a myocardial infarction based on history of smoking, blood cholesterol levels, and heart disease in the family were analytical studies. Studies may be retrospective or prospective. *Retrospective* studies analyze something that has already occurred. *Prospective* studies analyze factors affecting a situation as it evolves. When a number of babies were born with distinct physical deformities, hospital and prenatal records were studied to determine whether there were some factors common to the mothers' backgrounds which were found statistically more frequent in mothers of deformed babies versus a comparable group of mothers who delivered healthy babies. The drug thalidomide was found to be used by a significantly higher number of mothers delivering deformed babies than of mothers delivering normal babies. This was a retrospective study. Pregnant women who had taken thalidomide during pregnancy were identified and followed through delivery. A high proportion of the mothers delivered infants with this pattern of deformities. This was a prospective study.

Finally, an *experimental* approach is used to further investigate factors that have been implicated in analytical studies. The researcher sets up a situation that requires the research group to experience some specific situation and compares their reaction to that situation with a comparable control group which does not have that experience. For instance, studies were conducted to determine the effects of cigarette smoking on monkeys. One group of monkeys were forced to inhale cigarette smoke and another group had no contact with cigarette smoke. It was determined that a significantly high proportion of "smoking" monkeys developed lung cancer than "nonsmoking" monkeys. This was an experimental study.

The most common type of epidemiological research in which a nurse participates is an *epidemiological investigation*. Depending upon where the nurse works and the staffing pattern, the nurse may plan and implement the investigation or be a member of the team gathering the field data for the investigation while an epidemiologist or statistician may analyze the data.

Epidemiological investigations are primarily descriptive although some aspects of the analytical approach are used in determining differences among subgroups' experiences with an epidemic. An epidemiological investigation is often referred to as "shoe leather" epidemiology. Such an investigation seeks to determine the scope and cause of an epidemic in order to prevent additional cases and to determine control measures which would prevent another occurrence. This takes extensive field work, including interviewing those affected and those not affected, gathering specimens for laboratory analysis, and often, as the data is analyzed, returning to the community to gather additional specific information. Table 3-5 lists the steps of an epidemiological investigation and compares them with the steps of the scientific approach or research process. An epidemiological investigation begins with the determination that there is indeed an unusually high incidence of a health problem in a defined community (among a defined population).

Morbidity and Mortality Weekly Reports published by the Center for Disease Control in Atlanta, Georgia, summarizes reports of epidemiological investigations throughout the world, with emphasis on those in the United States. Although these are usually studies of reportable communicable diseases, the substantial investigations of Legionnaires' disease, cancer, and toxic shock syndrome have been reported.

The following is an example of a reported epidemiological investigation. In reviewing the report, apply the previously noted steps of an epidemiological investigation and answer the following questions: What was the initial outbreak reported (the identified problem)? Who was affected? Who was not? Where did it occur? When? What was the suspected cause (hypothesis)? What knowledge was this based on? What clinical data supported this hypothesis? What laboratory data supported this hypothesis? How was the initial problem revised as the investigation progressed? What mechanism of transmission was discovered—agent, avenue of escape, mode of conveyance, portal of entry, susceptible host? What environmental factors were of particular significance in the development of this outbreak? What control measures would stop the outbreak and would prevent further outbreaks with the company that prepared the spaghetti?

Staphylococcal Food Poisoning—Colorado
The Tri-County District Health Department (Denver) notified the Colorado Department of Health, July 28, 1976, of a staphylococcal food poisoning outbreak among employees of a Denver business related to a food vending machine. Eleven workers had become violently ill in the mid and late

TABLE 3-5. Comparison of Research Process with Epidemiological Investigation

RESEARCH PROCESS	EPIDEMIOLOGICAL INVESTIGATION
Define problem under investigation and purpose of study	Purpose—Determine occurrence and distribution
Develop tentative hypothesis(es)	Etiology—Associations
Review of literature/conceptual framework	Assessment of situation (outbreak)
	Problem identified
	Review of literature
	Knowledge of occurrence and distribution of disease and H-A-E Triad
Hypothesis(es)	Hypothesis (determination of possible causes)
Define variables	
Determine limitations	
Methodology	Approach to data collection
Sample from population	Population at risk
Instrument	Mechanism of transmission
Approach to data collection	
Collection of data	Collection of data
	Lab reports
	Attack rates
	Interviews
Analysis of data	Analysis of data
Descriptive—>statistics	Ratios/Rates—Biostatistics
Inferential	Interpretation of results
Interpretation of results	Definition of preventive and control measures, program planning
Future implications	

afternoon with nausea and vomiting. A few had diarrhea, but none had chills or fever. One patient was hospitalized. There was a statistically significant association between purchase of Greek spaghetti and illness (p = .001). Persons who ate other foods from the vending machine as well as some additional purchasers of Greek spaghetti did not become sick.

Because the catering firm supplying the hot food vending machines also serviced 15 other businesses at 29 locations in the greater Denver area, further inquiries were made to identify other affected persons. Three sick employees from 2 other businesses were found. They had typical symptoms of staphylococcal food poisoning.* All three had also eaten Greek spaghetti from hot food vending machines on July 28. One of the three was also hospitalized.

Because the vending machine company routinely prepared hot food items the day before sale, a questionnaire was given to food preparation employees about illness and food consumption at work on July 27. Two out of 10 evening employees reported illnesses characterized by abrupt onset of nausea and vomiting at 10:30 p.m. and lasting a few hours. They had eaten Greek spaghetti that evening at 6 p.m. Six of 8 other evening employees also ate Greek spaghetti but did not become ill with typical symptomatology. On the regular day shift, only 3 of 15 individuals had eaten Greek spaghetti; none of them had become ill.

Coagulasepositive Staphylococcus aureus, phage type 85, was cultured from the stool of the 2 hospitalized patients, the hands of 1 of the 5 foodhandlers preparing Greek spaghetti, the Greek spaghetti from 2 vending machines, and from the same brand of raw meat used in the Greek spaghetti.

S. aureus counts on Greek spaghetti recovered on July 28 at a temperature of 60 F from a vending machine at a Denver business were greater than a million organisms per gram. Greek spaghetti taken the same day from other vending machines at 160 F was culture negative. Other hot food items prepared on the same day taken from several machines on July 28 were also found to be contaminated with S. aureus, phage type 85, in smaller numbers. This same organism was also isolated from chili made the following day. Enterotoxin studies by the Food and Drug Administration laboratories found type D enterotoxin in samples of the implicated spaghetti taken the day of the outbreak from the machine at 160 F and in sam-

---

*Helpful information in discriminating between staphylococcal food poisoning and salmonella infection: Staphylococcal food poisoning: 1) incubation period 1-6 hours (usually 2-4); 2) type of food involved: wide variety—pastry, custard, salads, sandwich, meat and meat products; 3) source: ingestion of toxin from staph, carried in human skin infections; 4) symptoms: severe nausea, cramps, vomiting, often diarrhea and subnormal temperature. Salmonella: 1) incubation period 6-72 hours (usually 12-36); 2) type of foods involved: meat, egg, poultry products; 3) source: ingestion of organisms from contaminated food, usually due to inadequately cooked or handled food; 4) symptoms: sudden onset abdominal pain, diarrhea, nausea, vomiting and fever.[22]

ples taken from another unheated machine with a temperature of 60 F. However, all samples of staphylococcus type 85 were found to produce enterotoxin type A. Type D enterotoxin was also recovered from the chili samples taken the day of the outbreak at the food preparation area of the vending machine company.

The infected foodhandler had several blisters and a bandage on his hand when the cultures were taken. He handled the raw meat before cooking and, later in the day, helped portion cooked meat onto the spaghetti. In this food operation bare hands were routinely used for preparing cooked meat. An evaluation by Tri-County District Health Department sanitarians revealed that the central commissary refrigerator was inadequate to cool foods quickly. Many hot food items were found to be at a temperature favorable for growth of S. aureus as long as 8 hours.

This outbreak indicates that there was extensive cross-contamination because of poor foodhandling practices. The presence of type D enterotoxin suggests that the original toxin-producing organism was no longer recoverable at the time of the outbreak because other staphylococcal strains had overgrown the unidentified toxin-producing strain.

Reported by S. Johnson, M.D., J. Martyny, B.S., Tri-County Health Department, Denver; J. Humphreys, B.A., P. Mayfarth, B.A., J. Stambaugh, B.S., T. M. Vernon, MD, State Epidemiologists, Colorado Department of Health, in Colorado Disease Bulletin 4(41), 1976, Division of Microbiology, Food and Drug

In this example, the initial outbreak occurred at one business in Denver on July 28, 1976. A significant proportion of those eating Greek spaghetti became ill. Those who did not eat the spaghetti as well as those who ate other foods from the vending machine did not become ill. The suspected cause was the staphylococcal organism. This hypothesis was originally based on the signs and symptoms of those who became ill and on the time frame of the development of the signs and symptoms. As the investigation proceeded, cultures of food, hands of the food handler, and stool specimens of patients supported the initial hypothesis that S. aureus was the organism which caused the food poisoning.

The initial problem of an outbreak of S. aureus food poisoning in one business was revised as other businesses supplied by the food company and the personnel and procedures of the food company itself were investigated. The mode of transmission was as follows: The agent, S. aureus, began with Staph-infected hands which were draining live organisms into raw and cooked meat. This meat formed a culture in which the organisms could grow and produce toxins. The food provided the mode of conveyance, with ingestion of the contaminated food the portal of entry, and all persons eating the contaminated food became the susceptible hosts.

The method of preparation, handling, and storage of food by this company encouraged the development of such an outbreak. Control measures would include 1) destruction of all potentially contaminated food, 2) thorough cleaning with an appropriate bactericidal solution of all equipment involved in the preparation and storage of the food, 3) releasing the infected food handler from work until the individual was no longer contagious, 4) use of gloves in handling food, 5) education and routine inspection of foodhandlers to prevent infected workers from preparing or handling food, and 6) appropriate storage of foods to assure quick cooling and maintenance of foods at a temperature low enough to prevent bacterial growth.

Although it is not clear from this report who did the field investigation, in many smaller health departments the community health nurse would have done much of the interviewing and data collection.

The following story gives an example of how a school nurse might use the epidemiological investigation approach.

Story	Epidemiological Investigation Steps
In reviewing the health station records the nurse determines that during September 1, 1982, through October 31, 1982, there appears to be a high number (32) of children coming to the health station complaining of headaches, nausea, vague sense of not feeling well, and stomach aches.	Problem identified
In reviewing the previous years' records this pattern of symptoms had not occurred with this frequency during any other two-month period. The usual number of cases is 8 to 14.	Determination that incidence is of epidemic proportion
Because of the vagueness of the symptoms the nurse has a difficult time determining a possible diagnosis. She calls the health department to determine whether a communicable disease with this symptomotology is being reported throughout the community. It is not.	Establishing tentative hypotheses based on knowledge of possible causative agents
She also checks the records of other schools to determine whether this pattern is being reported in other schools. It is not.	Beginning data collection to test above hypotheses
In reviewing the health station records the nurse determines which students are being affected and which are not. Twenty are second graders from Room 201, which has 24 students. The remaining 12 students are scattered throughout the school in no discernible pattern. The	Determining the *who*

nurse notes a number of the same children from Room 201 have reported the symptoms two to three times. Therefore, what appears to be an attack rate of 80 percent is not substantiated.

The school nurse visits the class and asks the teacher her experiences with the children. The teacher indicates some children have complained of similar vague symptoms which were not severe enough to send the child to the health station. The teacher identifies these students; some have been to the health station, others have not.

Determining the *where*

In discussions with the teacher and reviewing the health station records, the nurse discerns a pattern of time of reporting these symptoms (between 10:30 AM and 12 noon). There is no identifiable pattern of time for the other 12 cases.

Determining the *when*

The school nurse decides to observe the class from 10 AM to 12 noon. She notes the class immediately breaks into three smaller reading groups of about eight children each. These groups are in different parts of the room and last for about 45 minutes. According to the teacher this is a change in method from the previous year. The nurse checks the list of students in the various groups against her list of students reporting symptoms and those not. Six of the eleven students reporting symptoms are in the reading group at the back left corner of the classroom. In observing this area the nurse notes it is furthest from the windows. She also notes the lighting in the classroom is structured for regular classroom rows of seats facing the front of the room.

Continued data collection and analysis

Knowing that the signs and symptoms of eye strain are similar to those reported by the students, the school nurse obtains from the health department an instrument to read the amount of light in this area. She then checks these readings against the standards required for schools

Hypothesis based on knowledge of possible causative agent

Data collection and analysis

for areas where children will be doing close work and determines the lighting is deficient for this area during this time of day.

Interpretation of results

The school nurse writes up her findings and presents them to the teacher and principal with recommendations for correcting this problem.

Recommendation of preventive and control measures

REFERENCES

1. LEAVELL, H AND CLARK EG: *Preventive Medicine for the Doctor in His Community.* McGraw-Hill, New York, 1965, p 39.

2. Ibid, p 40.

3. Ibid, p 40.

4. Ibid, pp 16–28.

5. SUSSER, M: *Causal Thinking in the Health Sciences: Concepts and Strategies of Epidemiology.* Oxford University Press, New York, 1973, p 3 (italics ours).

6. LITIENFIELD, A AND GIFFORD, A: *Chronic Disease and Public Health.* Johns Hopkins Press, Baltimore, 1966.

7. LEAVELL AND CLARK, op cit, pp 42–43.

8. US DEPARTMENT OF HEALTH, EDUCATION AND WELFARE: *Healthy People.* The Surgeon General's Report on Health Promotion and Disease Prevention. PHS Publication #79-550717, Washington, DC, 1979, p viii.

9. BLUM, HL: *Planning for Health.* Human Sciences Press, New York, 1974, p 622.

10. SUSSER, op cit, p 4.

11. DEVER, GEA: *Community Health Analysis: A Holistic Approach.* Aspen, Germantown, MD, 1980, p 20.

12. LEAVELL AND CLARK, op cit, p 95.

13. FRIEDMAN, G: *Primer of Epidemiology.* McGraw-Hill, New York, 1974, pp 11–12.

14. US DEPARTMENT OF HEALTH, EDUCATION AND WELFARE, op cit, p 43.

15. FRIEDMAN, op cit, p 13.

16. US DEPARTMENT OF HEALTH, EDUCATION AND WELFARE, op cit, p 16.

17. Ibid, p 21.

18. Ibid, p 13.

19. Ibid, p 13.

20. DEVER, op cit, p 5.

21. FOX, J, HALL, C, ELVEBACK L: *Epidemiology: Man and Disease*. Macmillan, New York, 1972, p 63.

22. BENENSON, A (ED): *Control of Communicable Diseases in Man*. American Public Health Association, Washington, DC, 1980, pp 137–139, 299–303.

CHAPTER 4

DESCRIPTIVE APPROACH TO COMMUNITY ASSESSMENT

OBJECTIVES

THE LEARNER WILL

1. identify the term health as defined in the descriptive approach to community assessment.

2. recall the three areas involved in a descriptive community assessment.

3. compare philosophical foundations of the descriptive approach to Orem's concepts of self-care.

4. recognize the place for the descriptive approach in the Discovery Process.

5. differentiate between themes and issues.

6. assess a community using the Discovery Process.

The descriptive approach to community assessment is a method of gathering health data about a community by investigating the physical, sociocultural, and economic conditions which affect those within the community. The assessment phase is the first step of an operational activity for assisting with the resolution of health problems by using the strengths and abilities of the individuals within the community.

The basis for this type of assessment is a view of health as a total life process—continuous, dynamic, and influenced by internal and external forces that are of a physical, sociocultural, and economic nature.[1] Communities use skills to manage their life processes based on the availability of resources and the ability to influence the various forces. Identification of these factors can give direction for adapting to new modes of action for improved quality of life.

The descriptive approach has been perfected by James Kent and associates through the development of the Discovery Process. There are a number of similarities between this Discovery Process and Orem's nursing theory in terms of conceptual approach to clients.

NURSING THEORY APPLICATION

Dorothea Orem proposes that clients use their own unique styles to provide for health care according to their capabilities.[2] These are identified as self-care abilities. The ability for self-care is influenced by numerous internal and external factors which can include cultural orientation, economic conditions, geographic area, political influences, present health status, and available resources.

The definition of self-care includes the following presuppositions:

1. Self-care is a form of self-management.
2. Self-care is necessary for life itself, for health, for human development, and for general well-being.
3. Self-care and the care of dependents rest on the cultural attainments of social groups and on the educability of their individual members.[3]

Orem focuses on the patient as an individual, with the health team and significant others viewed as a helping system. If the community is viewed as a client or patient, then the nursing process can be applied to the community, beginning with a history and assessment. The idea of self-care can serve as a theoretical foundation for the descriptive community assessment. Orem's theory can be interpreted to state that any condition that impinges upon the ability of the community to meet its physical, sociocultural, or economic needs can be considered a health care demand. A self-care deficit exists when the health care demand is greater than the self-care ability. A nursing relationship exists when the self-care deficit is great enough to project the client into a state of social dependency.

Community assessment using the descriptive method to ascertain self-care deficits begins with an identification of self-care abilities and health demands. The community or neighborhood is considered the basic unit for assessment, planning, and action. The Foundation for Urban and Neighborhood Development (FUND), directed by James Kent, uses the descriptive approach to initiate the Discovery Process. They advocate that the process begin with a description of the means by which the people in a community employ survival and learning techniques to manage their everyday lives. The interactions of the members of the community are observed as they relate to environmental constraints, support systems, and each other. It is not possible to separate community activity from the environment. Each modifies the other to affect the community as a whole.

Kent's Discovery Process uses the theory of "informal networks," consisting of people who support each other in predictable ways and have a shared commitment to maintain and to enhance their quality of life.[4] Discovery of the formal and informal networks, how they function, and the content of their interaction helps identify the strengths and weaknesses of the community and leads to a definition of the issues that disrupt or impinge upon the quality of community life. This assessment then gives direction to a social action process for change which incorporates citizen participation by using the network system. The "process begins with an ability to identify and tie issues to specific networks, because social action processes must always be grounded to the concerns of individual citizens and their constantly changing environments."[5] Figure 4-1 illustrates Kent's view of citizen participation and the Discovery Process.

Before beginning the assessment, Brownlee[6] suggests two areas that should be explored. The first is the attitude of the community toward "being studied." This is particularly true if the community is unique, such as having a specific ethnic orientation. The second is the need for an identification of any rules or protocols that should be followed during your investigation. Key informant interviews may provide this information. Ignoring this preparatory step could result in lack of acceptance and inaccurate data.

The chosen community may be one that is considered familiar to the investigator or it may be an unknown entity. In either situation, the approach should be that of a "stranger" involved in discovering hitherto unknown data. The investigation lends itself well to some techniques used in an anthropological investigation or the phenomenological approach.[7] An effort should be made to erase all preconceived notions regarding the area. It is best not to research formal data about the community before starting the project. This can be done at a later time.

Initial perceptions should be on a personal basis, using all five senses of sight, hearing, touch, smell, and taste.[8] This is accomplished on foot and alone. Walking around the area allows time for the senses to absorb the atmosphere of the neighborhood. Being alone is important. If two or more people start the activ-

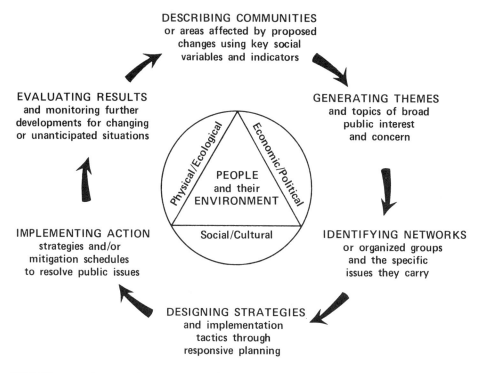

FIGURE 4-1. Diagram of Kent's view of citizen participation and the Discovery Process. (Redrawn from Health Care Strategic Management, November, 1983.)

ity together, it is only natural to share reactions, which will influence others' perceptions while they are occurring. A group of outsiders wandering around a close-knit neighborhood may cause suspicion and reticence to share. This may make it difficult to collect the correct information. If safety is a factor making it impractical for the assessment to be done alone, care should be taken so that observations are not shared with each other until the completion of this initial assessment.

The first walk through the neighborhood should not be hurried. Take time to observe. What is your first impression? Does it make you feel comfortable? Does it seem foreign to you? Sounds are significant. Is it noisy or quiet? What are the noises? Are they traffic, machinery, voices? Are they pleasant or distracting? Do you get the impression of purposeful activity? Odors can indicate industry, sanitation, cooking habits, or environmental problems. Try to get an overall impression while you are noting and absorbing the small details.

Physical Characteristics

Once the boundaries or limits to the community have been determined, physical features can be identified. The size and topographical features influence the character of the community. Cohesiveness, communication, and mobility may be affected by the size of the community. The geography of the area can influence the ability of the inhabitants to interact with each other. Cliffs, hills, mountains, rivers, and lakes are natural barriers which can divide a neighborhood. Artificial or man-made barriers include freeways, one-way arterials, railroad tracks, or anything that makes it difficult to cross in order to travel from one part of the community to the other. Tall buildings or large billboard signs, even though it might be easy to pass around or through them, sometimes act as visual or psychological deterrents to communication.

These same characteristics may well be the ones that serve to identify the boundaries of a community. The manner in which they influence transportation within the area and to the outside should be noted. Natural pathways used by the people as they travel to shopping or social congregation areas need to be identified. Modes and availability of transportation should be noted.

Climate affects the life style of the community. Housing, clothing, food, occupation, and the methods for adapting to the constraints imposed by severe fluctuations in climate can be assessed by direct observation or through discussions with the residents. The particular period in which the investigation is taking place may not give the entire picture of conditions throughout the year.

Vegetation is influenced by climate but can be an indicator of additional factors as well. It can inform the careful observer of the relative age of the district by the size of the trees and shrubs. Their condition may communicate a pride in the neighborhood, social or economic constraints, or a feeling of neglect and dissatisfaction. Cultural influences can be recognized by the nature and variety of vegetation. When economic conditions make growing vegetables a necessity, lawns may be replaced by a garden plot. Some communities have protested increasing water rates by discontinuing outside watering, or a water shortage may have made it impossible to irrigate.

The buildings and structures are good indicators of the "personality" of a community. The proportion of housing to industry, the type of housing—single family, multifamily, apartment or hotel—age and condition of housing are all economic and social indexes of living styles and possible health care demands. Communities pass through developmental stages similar to human growth and development. There is a growing phase, a stationary phase, and a deteriorating phase. The death of an individual community takes place when some new type of activity takes over the space of that particular community. The periods of changing between one phase and another are known as transition phases. Age and conditions of housing are frequently the first indicators of a changing phase in a community. Evidence of recent improvements or lack of repair could signal the direction a neighborhood is taking.

Physical conditions of the community—including buildings, sidewalks, lights, streets, or any other structure—may reflect the attitudes of the residents toward their circumstances. They may also be the result of outside political or economic policy at the local, state, or federal level. A quick survey of adjacent communities might be helpful as a comparison.

Signs can be another indicator of the attitude of the community residents

---

toward each other and outsiders. The usual street signs to control traffic and to protect pedestrians are to be expected and their absence questioned. House signs such as "Beware of Dog," "No Peddlers Allowed" or "No Trespassing" may be seen occasionally in any neighborhood. A large number of such signs should prompt further investigation of the situation surrounding the particular need for posting them.

Additional features of the neighborhood that should not be overlooked are the following: 1) *Fences.* These are a way of staking a territorial claim. They can be very attractive and meet the need for privacy or they can be forbidding and threatening. 2) *Recreation and shopping.* There should be provision for various types of facilities within the boundaries of the community which are conveniently located and meet the needs of its members. 3) *Parks.* Many neighborhoods have legal requirements for certain amounts of land to be allocated for park usage based on a percentage of the people residing in the area. It should be accessible and appropriate to developmental needs as well as having aesthetic qualities. 4) *Traffic.* Parking, flow, type, age and condition of vehicles may give clues to the nature of the neighborhood. 5) *Industry.* The variety, size, type, and amount of business conducted within the boundaries of the community can have a great influence upon the nature of the community.

Assessing the physical characteristics of the community can present a good beginning perception of its nature. It also serves as a basis for an introduction to an investigation of the social and economic factors which may affect the community's health demands and ability for self-care.

Social Characteristics

The social characteristics of a community are defined by the people who comprise the community. Their relationships with each other, the surrounding communities, and the government are areas to be defined. These relationships are influenced by many factors, including their culture, habits, modes of communication, and daily routines.

It is critical to talk with the people residing in the community. FUND developers learned that an "open process, rather than a 'back door' approach (stay invisible and hope that people won't know what you are doing) insures healthy community participation."[9] In this way as many issues as possible are identified and documented for resolution. The old-fashioned attribute of "passing the time of day" in a casual manner is a skill that should be encouraged. Professionals tend to have an agenda of preconceived ideas and a list of items which need answers. Community health nurses often claim more information can be gained about a client during the period of socialization at the beginning of a home visit than at any other time during the working phase of the visit. Talking may occur while walking around the area exploring its physical environment. Engaging in a conversation with someone who is hand watering the front yard, weeding the garden, or waiting for a bus might be appropriate. This sort of interaction can initiate ideas for further investigation.

Time might be spent on a park or bus stop bench observing the *activity of the people*. A stop at an establishment patronized by residents for refreshment, nourishment, and social interaction could be helpful. Browsing in some of the local stores will present an opportunity for observation and conversation.

The following excerpts from one of the author's experience as a participant in a community assessment workshop illustrate the talking technique and the information which can be acquired in this fashion:

A gravel country road, barbed wire fence enclosing a pasture of sparsely growing grass for two horses, one government low-income single family dwelling and a cluster of abandoned, unfinished multi-family housing. Blue skies, spring sunshine, meadowlarks calling and a few far-off traffic sounds and voices.

I was participating in a descriptive community assessment on the Ute Indian Reservation. This was my assigned area and I was becoming anxious. I had just been transported to the site, informed of my boundaries and abandoned. As I stood there undecided about how to proceed the residents of the single-family house emerged through the front door, got into their car and drove off down the road the way I had come. Since they were the only humans visible to me, I wondered how I was going to engage in a conversation with anyone!

I walked slowly along the dusty road and stopped in front of the pasture fence. I thought I might at least be able to contribute some observations to the assessment. The two horses were unkempt with protruding ribs, droopy heads and half-closed eyes despite the feel of spring in the air. The mare had a swollen belly and I mentally noted two alternatives—pregnancy or worms.

I moved on to the unfinished apartments a block away. They were framed and had outside siding, rough flooring, and sheetrock on the interior walls. There were no doors or windows nor any signs of wiring and plumbing. The dust had settled in a heavy coating to indicate cessation of building activity for some period of time. There were no signs of anyone using the building for any sort of activity whatsoever. Not even any vandalism.

I turned the corner of the road and there right behind another wire fence was a well-tended vegetable garden. The carrots were up about two inches in lovely even rows. My first thought was one of guilt because I hadn't even planted my carrots yet. Then I remembered I lived about a 1000 miles north and it wasn't planting time for us yet.

As I advanced to get a better look at the garden, a small boy about 8 or 9 years came around an unpainted shed towards me. We exchanged greetings and I expressed admiration for the garden. He said his mother planted it but she wasn't here now—she had gone to the store with his sisters and his grandfather was taking care of him.

He invited me to share a wooden garden bench under a tree in the back yard. As I gratefully accepted, I noticed his curious black eyes fixed on a stenographic notebook I was clutching more for a security blanket than anything else. I remembered I had red and black felt pens and a pencil in my purse so I asked him if he would like to draw in the notebook.

It was a truly inspired thought! He smiled and nodded, examined the drawing instruments, chose the pencil and went right to work. He drew a galloping horse ridden by a man with a lighted cigarette hanging rakishly out of his mouth. The smoke from the cigarette swirled up to the sky in fancy spirals. He explained that this was a picture of his brother racing his horse at the last powwow. He said his family attended several powwows each year. Sometimes they were on other reservations many miles away. There were games, visiting, no school and he thought they were great fun. It sounded rather like a large combination picnic and family reunion.

Then he drew another picture of a man with a rifle and said the men in his family went hunting for deer in the fall. This led to stories of hunting and fishing and he described a fish he had caught. His third picture was of Sitting Bull and he used both the colored felt pens to get the decorations of feathers and beads just right. He announced that Sitting Bull was a very important person.

I was just about to ask for the story of Sitting Bull when an elderly man came out of the back door of their house and over to us. The boy told me with pride that this was his grandfather. We introduced ourselves and I displayed the pictures his grandson had drawn.

I realized my feeling of discomfort had completely disappeared. I was about to continue with our conversation when one of the other participants in the assessment activity came rushing across the road to remind me it was time to leave. Our ride back was departing in a few minutes.

I had gathered a great deal of data in a very short time. There was the possibility of a morning routine as evidenced by the disappearance of the mothers and small children around 10 AM. I also knew there was an extended family system, social gatherings for entertainment and recreation, supplements to purchased food through a home garden, hunting and fishing, a cultural heritage, and here in this back yard a gentle and loving family. Further investigation would be needed to find out if cigarette smoking was a possible health hazard to Indian youth. The condition of the abandoned apartment complex led me to believe respect for another's property was important.

The concept of defining the *social characteristics* of a community is very broad. The social assessment might begin by determining recruitment and settlement patterns or the means by which people chose jobs and a community in which to live. Factors influencing these patterns include recreational activities, possibilities for employment, the life style of the community, or supportive services. Each community is unique. An effort should be made to identify the individuality of the community.

The *culture* of the community is a primary influencing factor. There may be one cultural focus for the entire community because of ethnic identity, occupation, geographic location, or custom. It may be a diverse community with many cultures, or there can be many combinations or adaptations to the cultural focus of the area. Care must be taken to avoid judgments and stereotypes. Personal cultural biases which influence thinking and conclusions should be avoided. The fresh view of a "stranger" will be helpful again.

Identification of the *routines* of the community will help to ascertain the best times to investigate social interaction and can be useful in planning ways to assist with health care demands. There are many factors that may affect the routines of an area. A hot climate may make it more comfortable for activity to take place in the morning when it is cool and in the late afternoon when the sun goes down. In rural areas with no mail delivery the community routine may be focused on the arrival of the mail at the local post office. The occupations of the wage earners or industry in the area may influence the routines. In an agricultural community, the daily schedule may vary depending upon the progress of the crops. Free time for other activities is limited by the demands of the season. Those who maintain livestock are controlled in the morning and evening by the need to "do the chores." A manufacturing firm may have an around-the-clock schedule, resulting in various segments of the population with differing routines.

In a low-income metropolitan area there may be increased activity at the first of the month when the government assistance checks arrive. The ability for self-care may also increase or decrease in proportion to the skills of the recipients to make their income stretch from one pay period to the next. In a suburban area the routines of the day may be guided by the school schedule.

The *communication system* is another important aspect of the social structure of a community. *Gathering places* can be identified. These are often related to routines and close to *natural pathways*. If mail delivery at the post office determines a routine, the gathering place for social interaction may well be the post office or a restaurant nearby.

In a farming community during the winter season farmers often gather at a local coffee shop sometime around midmorning. The laundromat near an area with rental housing may be a place where mothers socialize while washing their clothes. It may be more difficult to observe the interactions of homemakers having coffee together at a neighborhood residence, but it may be possible to determine if there is a routine for gathering in a particular residential area. These gathering places are part of the communication network because they provide a place and participants for communicating. Two other common communication methods are the telephone and individual contacts. Listening carefully when conversing with residents may be helpful in identifying the favored method of communication.

Closely allied to the principle of gathering for social interaction is the concept of the *natural caretaker*. During crisis periods or times of anxiety community members may seek assistance from individuals they view as helpful. The "helpful" designation can be based on a variety of personal attributes assigned to the helper, including knowledge, caring, support, previous success with the system, tradition, or custom.

Individuals may also take on the caretaker role as a part of their life style. The waitress in an eating establishment who advises an elderly customer to have fruit for dessert rather than ice cream because she knows he is diabetic may be such a person. Care must be taken to differentiate between the natural caretaker and the opportunist (market caretaker) who assumes this role for personal or financial gain.

Communication, routines, and natural caretakers produce a social network system for self-help within the community. An impression of the coping mechanisms used to deal with health care demands begins to emerge. This can be called the process by which the community uses self-care abilities. Health care needs or demands will also begin to present themselves as the investigator tries to identify self-care abilities.

Economic Characteristics

Economic and social characteristics of the community are closely interrelated. Data regarding both may be gathered at the same time. Information about the economic characteristics of a community may come from many sources. Observation of the physical nature of the area may quickly reveal the primary *focus of employment*—industry, agriculture, recreation, or small business. Initial perceptions can be verified through conversations with the residents. Some influencing factors relative to employment or personal income and their effect on self-care abilities and health demands include 1) availability, 2) permanence or seasonal nature, 3) "absentee" ownership or delegated management, 4) community attitudes, and 5) local, state, and federal controls, such as laws and/or policies.

Other factors that may be assessed relating to the individual workers that comprise the laboring population could include any changes in size or characteristics of the employment pool, the local labor supply, the mix of the population of those employed, and the management and wage structure.[10]

Power in a community frequently rests with those individuals who control the economy or finances. A group of nursing students investigating a deteriorating neighborhood using the descriptive method approached the manager of the nearest bank and asked him who he thought was the "power" in the community they were assessing. His answer was quite simple and straightforward. "I am," he said. Further inquiry revealed the city development plans projected industrial zoning for this primarily residential area. He was refusing requests for home improvement financing from anyone living there (an action sometimes referred to as *red lining*). Community efforts to upgrade living conditions were effectively frustrated. People were moving out of the area. He anticipated the properties would soon become available for industrial development.

Individual or small group *perceptions of the economic forces* within a community must be assessed as well as the broader economic influences. The ability to pay for services directly, through insurance, or via tax-supported programs is the present criteria in the United States by which health services are usually dispensed. Accessibility and availability of services are influenced by multiple economic factors.

Discussion of finances can be a forbidden topic because of cultural norms. This is true for the investigator as well as for those being investigated. The topic may be difficult to approach and may require some diplomacy on the part of the one seeking information. When lack of money is the cause for stress or precipitates a crisis situation, particularly when it affects the ability to meet the basic needs of life, the community may be more open to exploration of the problem.

Clues to economic conditions include prices in grocery stores compared with those in stores in other areas, signs about food stamp rules and regulations, check-cashing policies, and attitudes of clerks toward customers. Conversations with individuals frequently gravitate toward their state of health. It may be appropriate to discuss the current cost of illness and how it is financed.

Collating the Data

The Discovery Process adapts itself to an individual or group community assessment. When a group undertakes the process, participants may wish to divide the chosen geographic area into smaller units so that each individual will be investigating independently. Immediately after each session in the community, time should be allocated to jot down impressions as they come to mind. Journals, maps, or worksheets are useful for recording notes to assist the memory. It is not necessary to have these descriptive statements in any particular order or sequence. If there is more than one investigator, this is the appropriate time to share all the collected information with others in the group.

An effective process for group sharing is to appoint a recorder who writes all the thoughts and impressions on a blackboard or large sheets of newsprint. As the notations accumulate, clusters of related descriptions will begin to appear. These clusters can be called categories or themes.[11] In this instance, themes are "broad topics of public interest or concern. Themes cannot be acted upon directly, but focus the describer to pursue the identification of issues."[12]

An issue is a subject of widespread public discussion or interest. Issues are expressed desires of a specific network or group that can be acted upon at various stages of implementation development.[13] For example, expressions of dissatisfaction with public transportation may be identified as a theme from a group of descriptions which include conversations with people waiting for a bus, observations of only a single bus stop in the area, and reports of missed appointments and poor attendance at clinics or community centers because of transportation problems. An issue may be a proposed reduction in bus services or an increase in bus fares.

Themes help identify issues related to self-care deficits and health demands of the community. Networks transport the specific issues through the community. Networks identify the issues and are the means for implementing change. Therefore, it is important that networks and issues be described simultaneously.[14] Together they form the basis for determining problems and setting priorities for action. This approach results in a needs identification from the client's perspective. Just as effective nursing care of an individual or family requires client involvement, this method encourages community involvement.

REFERENCES

1. KENT, J: *A descriptive approach to community.* In: *Five Years of Cooperation to Improve Curricula in Western Schools of Nursing.* Western Interstate Commission for Higher Education, Boulder, CO, March, 1972.

2. OREM, DE: *Nursing: Concepts of Practice,* ed 2. McGraw-Hill, New York, 1980.

3. Ibid, p 22.

4. "The Use of Informal Social Networks in Natural Geographic Units as a Communication Method for Disaster Preparedness and Response." Unpublished research proposal, Foundation for Urban and Neighborhood Development (FUND), Denver, CO, 1983, p 9.

5. Ibid, p 10.

6. BROWNLEE, AT: *Community, Culture and Care.* CV Mosby, St Louis, 1978.

7. OILER, C: *The phenomenological approach in nursing research.* Nurs Res 31 (3): 178, 1982.

8. BAYER, M: *Community diagnosis—through sense, sight and sound.* Nurs Outlook 21(11):712, 1973.

9. *FUND News Release.* FUND, Denver, CO, 1982, p 1.

10. *Social-Resource Management Process.* FUND, Denver, CO, 1981.

11. *Discovery Process Training Handbook.* FUND, Denver, CO, May 1978.

12. *Op cit,* Unpublished Research Grant Proposal, FUND, 1983, p 12.

13. Ibid, p 10.

14. Ibid, p 12.

CHAPTER 5

SYSTEMS APPROACH TO COMMUNITY ASSESSMENT

OBJECTIVES

THE LEARNER WILL

1. describe the processes of input, throughput, and output of a given community.

2. identify possible negative and positive feedbacks into a system.

3. apply the concepts of systems theory in describing a community.

THE COMMUNITY SYSTEM

Systems theory provides an approach to delineating a specific community and to organizing assessment data into a meaningful format for decision making, priority setting, and program planning. In the process of defining a community to be assessed, the nurse determines who is to be included (the people or population) within what environmental perimeters. Through this process, the nurse identifies the living system which will become the focus of the assessment and establishes its boundaries; for example, who and what is within the system and what then forms its external environment. The area and people excluded by the boundaries are said to be outside the system and form the suprasystem. The defined system functions within the suprasystem. For instance, if the nurse chooses to define a community primarily on the basis of space (for example, a county), then the county lines become the boundaries which establish the people and environment within them as a system and separate them from the larger or suprasystem around it (for example, the state). The component parts of the system that make up the community are known as subsystems. The community system's components or subsystems can be separately identified, defined, assessed, and categorized.

Although a community is dissectable into its component parts (individuals, families, industries, service agencies), it is a whole—an entity—in itself. This entity relates to the surrounding larger community and is often dependent upon it for providing some aspect of the functions a community must perform. For instance, New York City has an identity of its own. Like other large cities, it cannot produce all the goods and services required to sustain its population. It must depend upon the larger suprasystem for food supplies. What the community of New York City does provide is a method for obtaining those goods and services which are not produced within its boundaries. Because of this exchange between the community and its suprasystem, a community is considered an open system. Just as the system (the community) is interacting constantly with the larger system within which it exists, the subsystems exist in dynamic interaction within the system and its environment. Demographic, epidemiological, environmental, and resource analysis data describe the structure of the subsystems of the community related to health status and quantity or quality of these subsystems. The processes occurring within the community may be determined through key informant interviews, surveys, and open forums which provide attitudes, values, perceptions of the community, and the interrelationships or patterns of interaction among subsystems which occur within the system. Observation and descriptive assessment further assist the nurse in determining both the structure and the interaction among its component parts which form the life processes occurring within the system. It is through the analysis of the relationships among the component parts of a system, its environment, and the suprasystem that the health status of the community may be determined, its health needs and resources identified, priorities determined, programs planned, and program impact estimated and evaluated.

CONCEPTS USED IN ASSESSING A COMMUNITY SYSTEM

An open system is constantly in the process of responding to internal and external stimuli and attempting to maintain a sense of balance or equilibrium. Because this state of equilibrium is not a static state, it has been referred to as a homeodynamic state or homeokinesis. In Chapter 1 the term communeokinesis was coined to refer to this same process within a community. The dynamic process used by the community to seek to maintain communeokinesis may be understood through application of concepts inherent in systems theory.

The flow of information and pattern of activity are important aspects of the functioning of a community. These are assessed when analyzing interactions among components of the community and the community and its external suprasystem. These interactions occur at the boundaries of each system: subsystems with subsystems, subsystems with the system, and the system with the suprasystem. These contact points are referred to as interfaces. The food distribution truck of a national chain store making a delivery to a local grocery store is an example of the interface between the system and the suprasystem. It is at these points of interface where change and/or conflict may occur.

Boundaries serve to maintain the integrity of the system just as the skin or integumentary system does for the human body. Boundaries do not necessarily have to be spatial characteristics such as rivers, mountains, and walls. They may be intangibles, such as socioeconomic status, culture, values, expectations, and policies. To a community health nurse in a well-child clinic in Chicago, it became obvious that mothers of children living three blocks away were not bringing their children to the clinic because these mothers were Puerto Rican and they would have to cross an invisible barrier separating their community from the black neighborhood in which the clinic was located. Boundaries control the flow of exchange into and out of the system. These exchanges are in the form of matter, energy, or information.

This exchange, when directed toward the system from the suprasystem, is termed *input*. The flow of migrant workers for the apple harvest or of college students into Fort Lauderdale at spring break becomes input into the community. The exchange across a systems boundary directed from the system to the suprasystem is defined as an *output*. When the workers leave the community with money in their pockets from wages earned, the harvest is exported from the community, or college students leave with new tans and new friendships, they become outputs of that community. During the period of time these individuals are participating in the community and interacting with other subsystems within the community, the inputs are processed and output is developed. "Input processing" and "output development" are called *throughput*. At times, input such as a large influx of people can overwhelm the available services and resources of a community. Gillette, Wyoming, expanded from a small range town to an expanse of trailer courts filled with young families during the oil and uranium boom. Its services such as schools, sewage, and water facilities were hard pressed to keep pace with the increased demand. An extreme output can be devastating. Consider the ghost towns left behind with the loss of the main source of an economic base—for example, silver and gold in Colorado and the lack of water during the drought in the Midwest in the 1930s.

Some portion or aspect of the output or results of the throughput of the system is returned to the system. This is called *feedback*, and, diagramatically, the loop leaving as output and returning as input back into the system is known as a feedback loop. One can also speak of feedback within the system owing to the dynamic interaction among components within the system. Feedback may be referred to as positive feedback or negative feedback. It is important that these terms are used as defined within systems theory rather than confused with concepts of good and bad or plus and minus. Positive feedback tends to continue the disequilibrium within the system which requires further adaptation. For example, in responding to a natural disaster, a city's services budget is depleted, preventing a planned increase in road and safety signs. Negative feedback tends to return the system to a state of equilibrium; either to its original state or to a different level of functioning. The same response to this natural disaster clears roads, allowing resumption of traffic and normal transportation of people, goods, and services.

EXAMPLES OF THE SYSTEMS APPROACH

The two following examples illustrate the use of the systems approach in community assessment.

A storm moves across Kansas, causing a blizzard in Wichita, Kansas. When the city of Wichita is viewed as a community, this blizzard would be an input from the suprasystem. The community's response to this blizzard would be the throughputs. These would include 1) decisions made by individuals as to whether or not to drive as well as how they are able to drive in the snow, and 2) decisions made by governmental agencies, for example, to close schools, to get snow removal crews out, and to institute emergency procedures that discourage unnecessary travel. These actions may produce the following outputs—increased number of accidents and emergency room (ER) visits, decreased work and productivity, increased efforts to clear highways, emergency efforts to supply food to shut-ins, increased use of energy for home heating. Positive feedbacks into the community might include such things as temporary disturbance in economic balance both for the community as a whole and for the city budget, caused by costs entailed in dealing with the blizzard; possible reduction of other services to shift resources such as staffing shifts in hospitals to handle the ER; and reduction of police efforts other than for traffic control. Negative feedback might include pulling the community together and an increase in community identity or a sense of shared camaraderie as people help each other. Figure 5-1 depicts diagrammatically the flow of this process.

A second example might be more focused on the interaction of the community and decisions made by a particular subsystem, the health department. Review of birth certificates indicates an increased rate of premature births, primarily with teenage mothers. This increase might be viewed as an input into the community system. In response to this input, the public health department makes the following decisions: 1) to increase prenatal services, 2) to increase community health nursing visits to "at-risk" prenatals and premature infants, 3) to increase community education programs in an attempt to prevent continuing incidence of premature births. These decisions (throughputs) result in in-

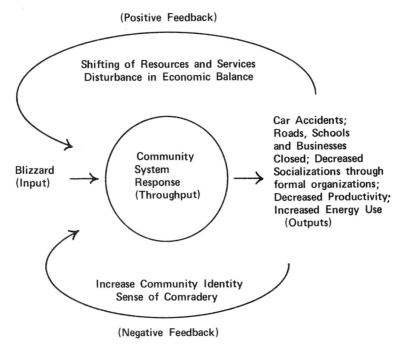

Shifting of Resources and Services
Disturbance in Economic Balance

Community
System
Response
(Throughput)

Blizzard
(Input)

Car Accidents;
Roads, Schools
and Businesses
Closed; Decreased
Socializations through
formal organizations;
Decreased Productivity;
Increased Energy Use
(Outputs)

Increase Community Identity
Sense of Comradery

(Negative Feedback)

FIGURE 5-1. Diagram of flow of input, throughput, output, and feedback in a community.

creased number of clinic locations and hours of service, increased assignment of community health nurses to these clinics and home visits, radio and television announcements, and community health nurses working with the schools and providing teaching and counseling sessions in the junior high and high schools. Negative feedback into the system from these outputs might include a decreased rate of premature births and an increased level of education regarding prenatal care and family planning in the community as a whole and the adolescent population in particular. Reduction of other services usually provided by the community health nurses, such as home visits to the elderly, and possibly increased costs or at least redistribution of resources from other services would be examples of positive feedback into the system (Fig. 5-2).

As can be seen by these examples, the process of throughput, its output, and the feedback this provides the system may have both beneficial and disruptive effects upon the system. Therefore, the decisions made or the processing of the input requires an analysis of as many of the potential implications as can be foreseen to determine the most effective response. This recognizes the fact that any action has the potential for both growth-producing and growth-inhibiting effects on the system. However, this is no different from giving a patient a medication. There are known side effects and complications of drugs which have to be balanced in the decision whether or not to use a specific drug for a specific patient. However, the more that is known about the patient and the contraindica-

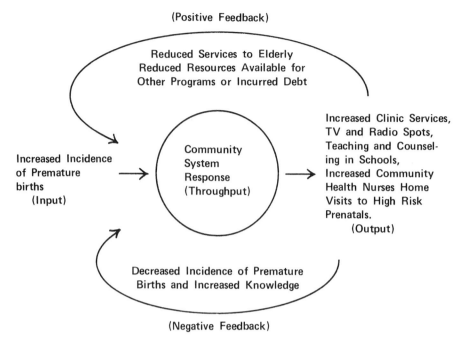

(Positive Feedback)

Reduced Services to Elderly
Reduced Resources Available for
Other Programs or Incurred Debt

Community
System
Response
(Throughput)

Increased Incidence
of Premature
births
(Input)

Increased Clinic Services,
TV and Radio Spots,
Teaching and Counsel-
ing in Schools,
Increased Community
Health Nurses Home
Visits to High Risk
Prenatals.
(Output)

Decreased Incidence of Premature
Births and Increased Knowledge

(Negative Feedback)

FIGURE 5-2. Diagram of flow of input, throughput, output, and feedback in a community.

tions of the drug, the more one reduces the risk and increases the benefit. This is exactly the same phenomenon which occurs with the community's attempts to deal with changes.

A final concept important in assessing a community from a systems approach is that of networks Networks are connecting links or channels within a living system. In a community they may be tangible, such as transportation routes and roads, or they may be intangible, such as communication networks, both formal and informal. Communities often include human networks through which key opinion formers affect decisions made within the community and control the type and flow of information. Using the family as an analogy, the nurse identifies who has the power to influence family decisions and works with and through that person; in a community, the nurse will learn to identify those who "get things done" or "prevent things from happening." Linkages among these people constitute human networks. The nurse's commonly accepted roles of advocate and coordinator attempt to create or to incorporate clients into such functional networks, and as facilitator, the nurse helps clients use available networks.

CHAPTER 6

ADAPTATION APPROACH TO COMMUNITY ASSESSMENT

OBJECTIVES

THE LEARNER WILL

1. recognize the community client as an adaptive system.

2. use Roy's Adaptation Model of nursing applied to a community to

   a. identify two major subsystems.

   b. recall three types of stimuli affecting environmental change.

   c. identify adaptive modes of a community.

3. determine the adaptive level of a sample community.

The concept of *adaptation* can be useful as a means of assessing the health needs of a community. There is an overwhelming amount of literature related to the content and process of adaptation. The most relevant adaptation model developed for nursing practice is Sister Callista Roy's[1] Adaptation Model of nursing. Using this model, the community health professional focuses on the community as an adaptive system. It has been identified that a community is considered to be a client or entity which can be viewed holistically—that its whole is greater than the sum of its parts. This community or client is considered a system existing within a larger environment.

Roy[2] includes two subsystems within the client system. These are the *regulator* and *cognator* systems. When there is a threat to the integrity of the system, the regulator system reacts to maintain homeokinesis or, in this instance, communeokinesis. In times of economic recession when members of a community have difficulty sustaining their means of livelihood, there may be an increase in volunteer activity and charitable contributions. Increase in criminal activity sometimes accompanies economic decline. The communication media become more active in alerting the community to dangers and suggest means to prevent criminal acts. There may be increased efforts to enlarge the linkage with other systems to provide or to supplement economic support. All these are examples of the regulator system's efforts to maintain a balance which allows the community to continue to function.

In a discussion of the community, the cognator system can be described as the community's sense of awareness and its ability to take deliberate group action. The cognator system is functioning when a large percentage of the population vote on a particular issue that affects the community. It can best be described in a negative way. When the cognator system is ineffective, there can be a lack of awareness of health disorders. The community is unable to identify its goals, to select a means to meet goals, or to reach its selected goals.

The community system, including its subsystems, has a constant internal and external interactional activity. This interaction produces change. Response to change results in a process termed coping or adapting. The level of adaptation is the relationship between the amount of environmental change (both internal and external) and the coping response. If the client does not adapt at an appropriate level, a health problem exists. The system is not in balance and cannot maintain an optimum level of wellness.

DEGREE OF ENVIRONMENTAL CHANGE

Roy[3] identifies three types of stimuli that determine environmental change. They are 1) *focal*, or a specific causal factor; 2) *contextual*, or all additional stimuli; and 3) *residual*, or the individual characteristics of the client. Community reaction to the arrest or shooting of one of its members by the police can be used as an example to illustrate the variations in these stimuli. The focal stimulus is the arrest or shooting. The contextual stimuli are the circumstances in which the incident occurred, previous experiences of the residents with police, and/or the presence of an organization for approval or protest. Residual stimuli include the mood of the community, its culture and values, its socioeconomic situation, and a multitude of other factors which can be identified as its characteristics. The adaptive reaction of the community to such a circumstance may vary from a simple item in the local newspaper and positive comments regarding the efficiency of the police to mass protests and violence attracting national attention.

These three stimuli are all input into the community system. The degree of environmental change is dependent upon the strength and duration of the stimuli and their interaction with each other and the system as a whole.

COPING RESPONSE

When the system is viewed holistically, it is common practice to divide it into subsystems and view the needs of the client in terms of physiological, social, and psychological needs. Cultural and spiritual needs are frequently subsumed under social or psychological needs. This division is a convenience that assists in categorizing needs even though the system is still considered a whole. Threats to any of these needs produce a response by the entire system, called adaptation. Roy suggests four ways of adapting which she terms *modes of adaptation*. They include response to threats to the integrity of 1) physiological needs, 2) self concept, 3) role function, and 4) interdependence.[4] These four modes of adaptation include the physiologic, psychologic, and social functioning of an individual client. Similarly, the functions of a community—because they incorporate physiologic, psychologic, and social functions—can also be used to identify modes of adaptation in relation to a community. The response would be to any threat to the integrity of the community to meet its needs in the areas of 1) use of space, 2) means of livelihood, 3) goods and services, 4) protection, 5) education, 6) participation, and 7) linkage with other systems. Table 6-1 illustrates some examples of possible adaptation or coping responses related to community functions.

ADAPTATION LEVEL

The adaptation level represents the relationship between the degree of environmental change and the coping response. According to Roy,[5] stimuli produce regulator and cognator activities, allowing the system to respond to any one or more of the modes of adaptation. Each client has an "adaptive zone." Within the boundaries of this zone, the client adapts positively to stimuli and is able to maintain an optimal level of wellness. When the coping response is ineffective, inadequate, or overreactive in relation to the environmental change and falls outside the client's adaptive zone, intervention is indicated.

TABLE 6.1. Adaptation Reponses Related to Community Functions

COMMUNITY FUNCTION	STIMULI	ADAPTATION RESPONSE
1. Use of space	Student population in school too large.	Redistricting, new school construction.
2. Means of livelihood	Underemployed, low industrial tax base.	Creation of industrial areas, organize to attract new industry.
3. Goods and services	Midcity grocery stores utilized by elderly are expensive, inadequate. Better shopping areas in suburbs.	Special transportation systems to chain stores outside of neighborhood for shopping. Develop grocery coops for midcity residents.
4. Protection	Increased incidents of mugging and thievery in low-income housing units.	Increase police protection, form volunteer protective units, organize education and publicity regarding preventive practices.
5. Education	Large group of Asian emigrants settle in the community.	Resident sponsors for Asian families, special classes in English, citizenship, and job training. Community integration activities.
6. Participation	Isolation of elderly in downtown hotels.	Increased social activity through visits, hotel socials, and excursions.
7. Linkage with other systems	Difficulty in obtaining drugs for treatment of rare diseases.	Federal legislation to give tax exemptions to companies to encourage manufacturing such drugs.

Areas of assessment to determine the existence of an adaptation problem include

1. Stimuli—focal, contextual, residual
2. Subsystem activity—regulator, cognator
3. Adaptive mode
4. Adaptive level—effectiveness of coping response.

The following description employs Roy's concepts to assess a community. A small community in western Montana identified the need for a new classroom in their local school. The community also decided against asking for federal assistance or state funds or raising school taxes to finance the building project. They agreed that they would try to raise the money by fund-raising activities—if possible, a single, large, community effort. Investigation showed that there were no organized Fourth of July celebrations within a 100-mile radius of their community. A local farmer donated the use of his barn and surrounding fields. They planned and organized a parade, carnival, and barn dance with an Independence Day theme. The community volunteered their participation. Publicity in a nearby major metropolitan area and surrounding communities was effective. The results were enough money to finance the building of the classroom.

The focal stimulus in this situation was an increase in the population of school-age children, producing a need for an additional classroom. The contextual stimulus was the reluctance of the people to use government or tax funds. The residual stimuli were the independence and self-sufficiency of the population, past experiences with obtaining other funding sources, and a knowledge of the community spirit and enthusiasm of its members.

The environmental change was the decision to raise the money through a community activity. The regulator subsystem responded with the offer of the use of the land and barn and the volunteering of community members to plan and to organize. The cognator system was able to recognize the need, to identify and to set goals, and to reach the goal of enough money to build a classroom.

Several modes of adaptation were in effect. There was a threat to the integrity of the educational system. The primary coping response was the provision of an additional classroom. This primary response also included other coping responses, such as participation, social interaction, production of services (the money-raising event), use of space for the activity, and linkage with the outside to attract the public.

The adaptation level was well within the adaptive zone. The community effectively adapted to the situation and maintained its communeokinesis. If sufficient money had not been raised in the first effort, the adaptive response may have been repeated until the goal was achieved. If the community were unable to reach its goal, appraisal of the process from the initial decision to raise the money by volunteer community activity through to the end result would pinpoint the problem area or areas.

REFERENCES

1. ROY, SC AND ROBERTS, SL: *Theory Construction in Nursing: An Adaptation Model.* Prentice-Hall, Englewood Cliffs, NJ, 1981.
2. Ibid, pp 60–66.
3. Ibid, p 55.
4. Ibid, p 43.
5. Ibid, p 45.

CHAPTER 7

OTHER APPROACHES TO ASSESSMENT

OBJECTIVES

> **THE LEARNER WILL**
>
> 1. recognize the potential for application of other theoretical models to community assessment.
>
> 2. distinguish between two process-focused approaches to assess a community's functioning.
>
> 3. identify tools and guides for community assessment in current literature.

In addition to the concepts and theories previously discussed, many others could serve as a conceptual base for developing a format for community assessment. Nursing draws from a variety of disciplines to develop a base for practice. For instance, developmental theories are used in assessing individuals and in planning appropriate interventions. A developmental model for community assessment could be designed to include an assessment of change in relation to direction, stages or levels, progression, causal factors, and potentiality.[1] Problem

---

OTHER APPROACHES TO ASSESSMENT   **85**

areas could be identified in the development of a community and analyzed in relation to growth and maturation. It would then be possible to project plans for future progress.

Neuman has formulated a Health Care Systems model which can be used to study the response of a community to stressors. It includes the concept of primary, secondary, and tertiary prevention and can be well adapted to community assessment.[2]

Other nursing theorists frequently speak of the individual patient or client as the primary focus of their theory. The view of the community as a client or entity in itself makes it possible to use their theories as conceptual frameworks for assessment.

A number of disciplines have developed approaches to community assessment. These include sociology, anthropology, community mental health, and health care planning. Many assessment approaches combine elements from a variety of disciplines.

PROCESS-FOCUSED APPROACHES

Two primarily process-related approaches have been developed which help the nurse determine the community's ability to function effectively, its modes of interaction internally, and its relation to the larger society. Goeppinger and colleagues[3] at the University of Virginia recently developed a model for assessing community competence using eight conditions Cottrell views as essential for community competence. These conditions are

1. Commitment—the attachment members have for their community,
2. Self-other awareness and clarity of situational definitions—accuracy of members of the community's perceptions of their and others' identity and position on issues,
3. Articulateness—ability for stating views in relation to those held by others,
4. Effective communication—accurate transmission of information,
5. Conflict containment and accommodation—effective management of differences among community members,
6. Participation—community involvement,
7. Management of relations with the larger society—utilizing external resources and stimulating development of additional resources, and
8. Machinery for facilitating participant interaction and decision making—responsive procedures which facilitate interaction and decision making.[4]

According to Goeppinger, assessment of indicators and components of these competencies are used to help explain community behavior and to provide direction to the nurse whose goal is to assist the community to effectively deal with concerns which affect the well being of the community as an entity.

Other nursing groups have used Warren as a basis for community assessment. Warren[5] developed a typology for classifying neighborhoods. He appears to use the terms community and neighborhood interchangeably. He conceptualizes the community as an information-processing center whose functioning can be understood by assessing and analyzing three principles of organization: interaction, identity and connections.

1. Interaction—the patterns of interaction among the members of the neighborhood.
2. Identity—the way in which the members perceive the community and the degree of a sense of shared commonality.
3. Connections—the degree to which members of the community participate in activities outside the neighborhood which have a potential impact upon the neighborhood.

Warren[6] identifies six types of neighborhoods based on an assessment of these three qualities and of the interaction among them. These types are integral, parochial, diffuse, stepping-stone, transitory, and anomic. From this typology, Warren determined eight key characteristics which should be considered when selecting a strategy or combination of strategies useful to encourage community action on any given concern. He then suggests which strategies would be most effective to mobilize community action according to each key characteristic.

Both models focus on the community as an entity and assess its method of operation. These approaches are quite useful when combined with data from other assessment approaches which identify areas of health concern within the community because they add an important component which assists the nurse to adapt interventions to the specific community's method of functioning.

ASSESSMENT TOOLS AND GUIDES

Other authors have developed tools or guides for performing a community assessment. These generally incorporate select concepts of systems theory, focus on components of the definition of a community—a people, a place, and a social system, and are grounded in those ideas derived from the definition of community—its elements and functions.

The "Community Nursing Survey Guide," published by Tinkham and Voorhies[7] in their book "Community Health Nursing: Evaluation and Process, is probably the most comprehensive of these tools. This 14-page assessment guide focuses on a description of the community, its population, environment, health and illness patterns, communication, health resources, and offers an extensive assessment of community health nursing services.

Clemen and colleagues[8] have published a "Community Assessment Tool:

Overview of Its People, Environment, and System" in their book *Comprehensive Family and Community Health Nursing.* This eight-page guide provides for identification of strengths, potential needs, and problems related to the population and the environment. It includes an assessment of the systems through which services are provided and the dynamics of communication within the community and connecting it to the larger society.

Helvie[9] presents a 13-page "Community Nursing Assessment Guide" in his book *Community Health Nursing: Theory and Process.* This guide more heavily relies on systems theory in providing a format for describing the community and its various subsystems: economic, education, communication, political, religious, recreation, transportation, welfare, families, and health, including community health nursing services. He also provides for an assessment of community dynamics, exchanges with the nonhuman environment, and exchanges beyond the community.

In her *Community Health Nursing: Concepts and Practice,* Spradley[10] presents a brief three-page outline titled "Community Profile Inventory." This inventory focuses on data to be collected in relation to location, population, and social system. It identifies factors to be assessed, lists community health implications, community assessment questions, and information sources for each factor.

Elkins[11] presents a brief four-page "Guide for Community Assessment" in her *Community Health Nursing: Skills and Strategies* which identifies the basic information a community health nurse needs to know about the community within which the nurse works.

Friedmann's[12] recent community health nursing text recognizes the importance of community assessment and provides the following suggested areas for data collection—U.S. census, community services, community characteristics, population characteristics, health and illness patterns, and environmental influences.

A number of faculty groups teaching community health nursing have developed their own assessment guides to direct student learning experiences in community assessment. Rauckhorst and colleagues[13] at Lehmen College in New York City published a one-page "Community Assessment Guide" which is a topic outline of factors to be assessed under major headings of overall features, population characteristics, service facilities, and environmental/safety conditions. At the University of Rochester, Stein and Eigsti[14] published a one-page guide based on the Data Base Management System developed by Christianson. The "Categories for Recording Descriptive Community Data" outlines categories related to physical environment, social and behavioral factors, and government. Later in the term, students incorporate census tract data, vital statistics, and information from agency and community leaders into their assessment to determine community nursing diagnoses. Allor[15] at the University of Michigan, Ann Arbor, published a two-page "Community Profile" instrument which assists students to collect data, to weigh their implications for the community, and to draw conclusions regarding the following community components: community description, population characteristics, population facilities, environmental characteristics, and health characteristics, including health care resources.

Community mental health literature provides direction for need assessment and service evaluation. One example is the needs assessment instruments published by the National Institute of Mental Health in *Needs Assessment Approaches: Concepts and Methods.*[16] Risk-reduction literature includes studies and survey instruments used to determine high-risk groups. One example is the "Lifestyle Assessment Questionnaire" published by Faber and Reinhardt[17] in their book *Promoting Health through Risk Reduction.* These guides and surveys would serve as helpful resources for nurses wishing to use an established guide or to obtain a base from which to develop their own assessment instruments.

REFERENCES

1. RIEHL, JP AND ROY, C: *Conceptual Models for Nursing Practice.* Appleton–Century–Crofts, New York, 1974, p 56.

2. Ibid, pp 99–134.

3. GOEPPINGER, J, LASSITER, PG, WILCOX, B: *Community health is community competence.* Nurs Outlook, September/October, 1982, pp 464–467.

4. COTTRELL, LS: *The competent community.* In Kaplan BH, ET AL (EDS): *Further Explorations in Social Psychiatry.* Basic Books, New York, 1976, pp 195–209.

5. WARREN, D AND WARREN, R: *Six kinds of neighborhoods.* Psychology Today June 1975, pp 75–80.

6. Ibid.

7. TINKHAM, C AND VOORHIES, E: *Community Health Nursing: Evaluation and Process.* Appleton–Century–Crofts, New York, 1977, pp 277–290.

8. CLEMEN, SA, ET AL: *Comprehensive Family and Community Health Nursing.* McGraw-Hill, New York, 1981, pp 64–71.

9. HELVIE, C: *Community Health Nursing: Theory and Process.* Harper & Row, Philadelphia, 1981, pp 304–316.

10. SPRADLEY, BW: *Community Health Nursing: Concepts and Practice.* Little, Brown & Co, Boston, 1981, pp 367–369.

11. ELKINS, CP: *Community Health Nursing: Skills and Strategies.* Robert J. Brady, Bowie, MD, 1984, pp 48–52.

12. FRIEDMANN, ML: *Manual for Effective Community Health Nursing Practice.* Wadsworth, Belmont, CA, 1983, pp 18–29.

13. RAUCKHORST, L, ET AL: *Community and home assessment.* Journal of Gerontological Nursing 6: (6) 319, 1980. Or in SPRADLEY, B: *Readings in Community Health Nursing.* Little, Brown & Co, Boston, 1982, pp 154–165.

14. STEIN, KZ AND EIGSTI, DG: *Utilizing a community data base system with community health nursing students.* Journal of Nursing Education 21 (3): 26, 1972.

15. ALLOR, M: The "community profile." Journal of Nursing Education 22 (1) 12, 1983.

16. WARHEIT, G, ET AL: Needs Assessment Approaches: Concepts and Methods. National Institute of Mental Health, Rockville, MD, 1977, pp 107–135.

17. FABER, M AND REINHARDT A (EDS): Promoting Health Through Risk Reduction. Macmillan, New York, 1982, pp 207–238.

UNIT BIBLIOGRAPHY

ALLOR, M: The "community profile." Journal of Nursing Education 22(1):12, 1983.

BAYER, M: Community diagnosis—through sense, sight and sound. Nurs Outlook 21(11):712, November 1973.

BENENSON, A (ED): Control of Communicable Diseases in Man. APHA, Washington, DC, 1980.

BLUM, HL: Planning for Health. Human Sciences Press, New York, 1974.

BRADEN, CJ AND HERBAN, NL: Community Health: A Systems Approach. Appleton–Century–Crofts, New York, 1976.

BROWNLEE, AT: Community, Culture and Care. CV Mosby, St Louis, 1978.

CLEMEN, SA, ET AL: Comprehensive Family and Community Health Nursing. McGraw-Hill, New York, 1981.

COHEN, JB: Florence Nightingale. Sci Am 250:128, 1984. (This article concerns her extensive use of biostatistics.)

COTTRELL, LS: The competent community. In KAPLAN, BH, ET AL (EDS): Further Explorations in Social Psychiatry. Basic Books, New York, 1976.

DEVER, GE: Community Health Analysis: A Holistic Approach. Aspen, Germantown, MD, 1980.

Discovery Process Training Handbook, FUND, Denver, May 1978.

ELKINS, CP: Community Health Nursing: Skills and Strategies. Robert J. Brady, Bowie, MD, 1984.

FABER, M AND REINHARDT, A (EDS): Promoting Health Through Risk Reductions. Macmillan, New York, 1982.

FOX, J, HALL, C, ELVEBACK, L: Epidemiology: Man and Disease. Macmillan, New York, 1972.

FRIEDMAN, G: Primer of Epidemiology. McGraw-Hill, New York, 1974.

FRIEDMANN, ML: Manual for Effective Community Health Nursing Practice. Wadsworth, Belmont, CA, 1983.

GEORGE, JB: Nursing Theories. Prentice Hall, Englewood Cliffs, NJ, 1980.

GOEPPINGER, J, LASSITER, PG, WILCOX, B: Community health is community competence. Nurs Outlook, September/October, 1982, pp 464–467.

HALL, J AND WEAVER, B: *Distributive Nursing Practice: A Systems Approach to Community Health.* JB Lippincott, Philadelphia, 1977.

HANCHETT, E: *Community Health Assessment: A Conceptual Tool.* John Wiley & Sons, New York, 1979.

US DEPARTMENT OF HEALTH, EDUCATION, AND WELFARE: *Healthy People.* The Surgeon General's Report on Health Promotion and Disease Prevention. PHS Publication #79-550717, Washington, DC, 1979.

HELVIE, C: *Community Health Nursing: Theory and Practice.* Harper & Row, Philadelphia, 1981.

KENT, JA: *A descriptive approach to community.* In: *Five Years of Cooperation to Improve Curricula in Western Schools of Nursing.* Western Interstate Commission for Higher Education, Boulder, CO, 1972.

KENT, JA AND KENT, ST: *Environmental continuity: A social-geographic approach to structural change in lowering health care cost through elderly participation.* Health Care Strategic Management, November 1983.

LEAVELL, H AND CLARK, E: *Preventive Medicine for the Doctor in His Community.* McGraw-Hill, New York, 1965.

LITIENFIELD, A AND GIFFORD, A: *Chronic Disease and Public Health.* Johns Hopkins Press, Baltimore, 1966.

OREM, DE: *Nursing: Concepts of Practice,* ed 2. McGraw-Hill, New York, 1980.

RAUCKHORST, L, ET AL: *Community and home assessment.* Journal of Gerontological Nursing 6(6):319, 1980. Or in SPRADLEY, B: *Readings in Community Health Nursing.* Little, Brown & Co, Boston, 1982.

RIEHL, JP AND ROY, C: *Conceptual Models for Nursing Practice.* Appleton-Century-Crofts, New York, 1974.

ROY, SC AND ROBERTS, SL: *Theory Construction in Nursing: An Adaptation Model.* Prentice-Hall, Englewood Cliffs, NJ, 1981.

Social-Reference Management Process. FUND, Denver, 1981.

SPRADLEY, B: *Community Health Nursing: Concepts and Practice.* Little, Brown & Co, Boston, 1981.

STEIN, KZ AND EIGSTI, DG: *Utilizing a community data base system with community health nursing students.* Journal of Nursing Education. 21(3):26, 1972.

SUSSER, M: *Causal Thinking in the Health Sciences: Concepts and Strategies of Epidemiology.* Oxford University Press, New York, 1973.

TINKHAM, C AND VOORHIES, E: *Community Health Nursing: Evaluation and Process.* Appleton-Century-Crofts, New York, 1977.

WARHEIT, G, ET AL: *Needs Assessment Approaches: Concepts and Methods.* National Institute of Mental Health, Rockville, MD, 1977.

WARREN, D AND WARREN, R: *Six kinds of neighborhoods.* Psychology Today, June 1975.

UNIT 3

CLINICAL JUDGMENT

This unit deals with some of the clinical judgments nurses make when assessing a community. These include factors to be considered in choosing an approach or combination of approaches to community assessment, drawing inferences during data collection, developing community diagnoses, and determining their implications for nursing practice.

When a person arrives at the emergency room of a hospital, is admitted to a unit, or is referred to a visiting nurses association, the initial contacts made by the respective nurses include an assessment of the individual. The setting, the nature of the individual's presenting health problem(s), agency policies, time, economic limitations, the nurse's repertoire of skills, and conceptual approach all affect the assessment which will take place. What will be the nature and extent of assessment data collected? What procedures and techniques will be necessary? What systematic approach will be used in the collection and organization of the assessment data? And, finally, what is the meaning of the data being collected? All these questions are questions of clinical judgment.

CHAPTER 8

ISSUES IN SELECTION, COLLECTION, AND ANALYSIS

OBJECTIVES

THE LEARNER WILL

1. identify the variables that determine the choice of approach used in assessing a community.

2. recall the strengths and weaknesses of four different approaches to community assessment.

3. recognize issues in selection of relevant assessment data.

4. evaluate assessment data in relation to sources, sample, validity, and accuracy.

CHOICE OF APPROACH

The idea that initiates the determination to conduct an assessment may range from the statement "Let's do a little study to see what the problem is" to the need for a comprehensive assessment of a community in order to plan programs as effectively as possible. The decision regarding the purpose of the assessment may originate with an individual or an administrative directive, or it may be generated by the community itself.

The purpose of a community assessment is to give direction for the choice of a framework for assessing community health needs. Purposes include needs identification, problem clarification, desire analysis, resource identification, and resource utilization.

There are many additional factors which can influence the selection of a specific approach or combination of approaches. A major consideration can be the resources available to those who are going to be involved in the assessment. These resources include personnel, time, finances, access to data, and the political-social-cultural atmosphere surrounding the situation.

The size or scope of the assessment influences the need for resources. The individual community health nurse with a new assignment to a well-child clinic may wish to assess the families who attend the clinic to better understand the nature of their health problems. The community would be comprised of those clients participating in the well-child clinic. Some of this information could be gathered during the client visits to the clinic, through personal interviews, review of their records, and discussion with the clinic personnel who work with the clients. Further data might be obtained from the vital statistics section of the local health department for the area that the well-child clinic serves. If follow-up home visits are indicated as part of the routine for clinic participation, additional information would be obtained as the nurse made these visits. In this instance, the data are available within the working situation. The resources necessary to carry out the assessment would be minimal. The nurse can collect much of the information while performing normal nursing functions. The time allocated to plan the assessment and to organize and to analyze the data would be the financial investment of the employer toward an assessment such as this.

If an assessment on a large scale is planned, there may be a number of steps required before resources can be determined. The boundaries of the community must be estimated to give an idea of the size of the project even though the projected boundaries may change as the assessment progresses. Establishment of boundaries gives definition to the geographic size and the number of people within the community to be assessed. In the preceding example, the boundary of the community was identified simply as the families who attend the well-child clinic. It may be more difficult to determine the exact area encompassing a migrant worker population or those unemployed as the result of the closure of a particular factory.

The size and type of community then suggests the number of people to be involved in the assessment and the qualifications of the investigators that would make them most suited to conduct the assessment. Nurses, environmental health specialists, epidemiologists, laboratory personnel, mental health practitioners, sociologists, and community members may all need to participate or at least to contribute in some way to the development of the assessment approach.

Some decisions will need to be made regarding budgetary restrictions.

Limits could be set regarding the number of personnel and the time frame the assessment might encompass. If there are no plans to hire people specifically for the assessment task, the amount of time it would draw the personnel away from their regular duties should also be calculated as a financial factor. These decisions will be influenced by the structure and size of the agency or the situation.

Access to data and the political-social-cultural climate have also been cited as resource considerations. Data may have already been collected in some areas related to the assessment. It should be determined if that information is relevant and available. State and federal studies may take some time and effort to obtain. Local studies may be more accessible.

The individual or group who initiates the idea for an assessment must gain the approval and support of those who are going to provide the resources to carry out the investigation. In the work situation, this may move directionally up toward administrative superiors or down toward the staff. A community-initiated assessment request may already have the support of its leaders or the community power structure. If not, failure to gain such support may ultimately present obstacles in the progress of the activity. Because carrying out the assessment involves the cooperation of the population within the community, an effort to establish and to maintain goodwill is necessary.

When the purpose of the assessment and an indication of the resources for carrying out the activity have been determined, then a framework for assessment can be proposed. The chosen approach or framework may be dependent upon the resource allocation and the kind of information needed to complete the assessment. The framework may suggest the need for a participant with a particular expertise. It is also possible the appointment of an individual with certain qualifications or background to the assessment group may give direction to the choice of approach.

Consideration should be given to the philosophy of the institution or agency providing the resources and to whom the material is to be presented. Nursing personnel in a hospital using a specific nursing theory as a basis for nursing practice might more readily understand and accept an assessment based on that particular nursing theory. Health departments have an extensive background in disease detection and prevention. These agencies might be more open to an assessment based on the epidemiological approach.

It is important to consider the audience in choosing a framework for assessment. Not only does the assessment activity as directed by a specific approach need to be accepted by the participants in that activity, but the type of material collected must also be acceptable to the group for whom it is intended. If the purpose of the assessment is to obtain information for a grant proposal, it is necessary to include all the information requested according to the guidelines of the grant. For example, baccalaureate nursing students with community assessment assignments are always eager to identify exactly what type of approach is more agreeable to the faculty audience. Presenting the material to a group with a business background may require content with emphasis on economic data. Community leaders and politicians may be very interested in problems that affect the feelings and attitudes of their constituents.

An analysis of the kind of information desired can also indicate an approach. If the intent is to obtain all the factual data contained within a specified area, such as *identification* of community resources, a simple survey may be all that is necessary. An assessment of community resource *utilization* broadens the focus to include not only the resources available but also the interaction of the components of the community among themselves and with their environment in relation to community resources. A process-oriented approach is more appropriate under these circumstances.

Sometimes the community to be assessed has already been the recipient of similar activities. The intent of the assessment is to confirm previous data or to obtain information that has not been elicited before. For validation purposes, the same approach may be repeated. A different approach may also validate previously collected data. A different approach can view the same material in a different way and lead to the same or differing conclusions regarding the information collected.

STRENGTHS AND WEAKNESSES OF APPROACHES

Each conceptual approach to community assessment has strengths and weaknesses. It is important that the nurse take this into consideration when designing a community assessment format.

Epidemiological Approach

The epidemiological approach to community assessment refers to a number of related approaches. They all have in common, however, the use of statistics to describe the health status of a population. The nurse may analyze statistics already developed about the community under study or use statistics in an epidemiological investigation.

An epidemiological investigation is particularly useful when the nurse identifies an unexpected occurrence of some health disorder. This approach is usually used to follow up on a recognized problem to determine its source and to identify a method of preventing further instances of the health problem in a given population. It may be used regardless of the nature of the health disorder being experienced in that population. An epidemiological investigation requires a focus and, therefore, is not the most useful approach when the nurse is initiating a general assessment. It might be likened to a chief-complaint-oriented assessment rather than a screening assessment with an individual client.

An epidemiological investigation can be performed at a relatively simple level by a nurse with a fairly prescribed population, or it may be performed on a nationwide scale with a high degree of expertise, such as the Center for Disease Control's investigation of Legionnaires disease and toxic shock syndrome.

This approach requires the ability to calculate and to interpret rates and to use the scientific method. It provides measurable data which are valuable in supporting the investigator's conclusions. However, such statistics are useful only when interpreted accurately and are meaningful to the audience to which they are presented.

Statistical data previously obtained about a community, such as morbidity and mortality statistics, and demographic data provide a general description of the population, its characteristics, and health problems. These data might be likened to an individual client's health history and description of basic characteristics. Such statistical information about a community gives a basis for comparisons with "norms" or outside standards, as well as a comparison with previous baseline data from the same community. Demographic data coupled with a knowledge of the implications of risk factors for developing certain diseases provide a projection of potential health problems and a basis for categorizing these problems in terms of the priority of the problem.

An epidemiological investigation does not provide information on the community's perception of the problem or its values and processes for decision making. It can indicate possible sources of the problem and points of intervention but not the political milieu within which decisions will be made, nor can it determine the likelihood of acceptability of alternative solutions. This may be likened to knowing the physical assessment data which indicate that a client is hypertensive owing to atherosclerosis but not having any data on the client's life style and values, which so strongly influence the patient's compliance with the medical regimen that may be ordered.

A weakness of this approach is that epidemiological data do not assist the nurse to determine the strengths of the community; nor does it provide a holistic view of the client. Therefore, the epidemiological investigation itself should be used once a health concern is identified in order to determine the occurrence and distribution of the problem, its source(s), and possible alternative interventions. Vital statistics and demographic data make valuable contributions to the determination of the health status of the community and potential health concerns and health care needs. The addition of other approaches will be necessary to provide a basis for determining appropriate interventions.

Descriptive Approach

The major advantages of the descriptive approach to community assessment are its holistic orientation and its focus on the community as it exists for its residents. Just as the community health nurse considers the home visit to be the foundation of practice, the descriptive approach serves much the same purpose. Both allow assessment in the environment in which the client is functioning. When the investigator gathers assessment data by observation and discussion in a nonjudgmental manner, the community is able to give input in its own natural style.

Strengths of the community as well as its problems can be discovered. This information is very important as a basis for the process of implementing action. Rehabilitation after a heart attack cannot succeed without the cooperation of the heart attack victim and the family. Consideration must be given to psychological, social, cultural, and spiritual orientation, and wishes of the client as well as the physical condition. This is also true of the community client.

The descriptive approach is flexible. It can be used by a person as an orientation to the community. The health care worker assigned to a new area may want to spend some time using this approach before beginning practice in the area. Information derived from this type of assessment can give direction concerning type and location of goal-oriented projects, such as a new health clinic or other health service in a community. On a larger scale, it can be used as the basis for comprehensive health planning for an entire geographic area.

The ability to be an alert, objective observer is the major requirement of the descriptive approach investigator. This allows the coordinator of the activity to draw participants from a variety of backgrounds and interests. Extensive academic or professional preparation need not be prerequisite. This can be advantageous if personnel resources are limited. The inclusion of a variety of participants adds diversity to the data collected and greater opportunity to insure validity of the data.

The major weakness of this approach also has to do with the investigative participants. In order for the process to succeed, each investigator must be open to accepting the input in an objective way without preconceived attitudes and values. An effort must be made to avoid value judgments. Although the odor of sagebrush may be pleasant to some, it is disagreeable to others; its aromatic presence can still be noted.

A group activity that includes several investigators allows for validation of information. This can be expensive in terms of salaried personnel. The investigation may require a considerable period of time if any true sense of community life style is to be obtained. The time frame is also important if the community changes seasonally. Activities and health problems of residents in a rural agricultural community, for example, may be very different as the season progresses. Allocation of adequate and appropriate time for the assessment is necessary. Financial considerations or a problem situation requiring immediate attention may not allow for this kind of time investment. In the long run, however, it may be more expensive not to perform a comprehensive assessment.

Systems Approach

The greatest strength of the systems approach is that it assists the nurse to analyze the way a community functions as a unit and how it relates to its environment and the rest of society. It is a process-oriented assessment. As such it provides a context within which to organize and to analyze assessment data rather than techniques of data collection. Many of the concepts basic to systems theory are used in business, health care, and education and may be familiar to the audience to which the assessment is presented. As is common with many theoretical approaches, systems theory has its own language, and that language often is not in such general use as the concepts to which the language refers. Therefore, the nurse must assure that the formal language of systems theory which helps the nurse conceptualize what is happening in the community does not overwhelm the intended audience. Because the systems approach focuses on the interrelatedness of aspects of the community, it is holistic and includes both strengths and problems. Its use requires knowledge of assessment data categories and assessment techniques to gather appropriate data regarding the client. Therefore, the nurse must use multiple sources and techniques with this approach.

Analysis of a community's response to a health concern provides the nurse with a perspective on the decision-making process within the community. Using such an approach when a health concern arises provides a mechanism for projecting alternative responses in the community and the potential impact each would have on the community and its surrounding environment. In this way the nurse is able to assist the community to solve problems and to determine the most appropriate action.

Adaptation Approach

Adaptation is based on systems theory and is process oriented. The product of such an assessment should result in a holistic view of the community and its surrounding environment. It concentrates on the functioning of the client in response to stimuli and is, therefore, humanistic in its approach. Past and present responses give direction for future action.

The greatest strength of the adaptation approach is its basis in the process of coping. This necessitates the investigation of the positive strengths of the community in order to determine gaps in the coping process and the presence of negative coping mechanisms. These strengths can be recognized and used in the planning and implementation stages, resulting in more effective programs. If a community relies on its church for spiritual and social sustenance, a food program or health clinic organized through the auspices of the church may be more successful than the use of an outside agency to administer such a program.

It has previously been suggested that the functions of the community should be the criteria for assessing modes of adaptation. Although effective functioning in all these areas can produce positive self-concept in relation to community, this category was not identified specifically for assessment. Roy includes self-concepts as one of the four modes of adaptation and, therefore, gives it equal status with physiological needs, role function, and interdependence.

Whether self-concept is subsumed within each category of the functions of a community, a separate category or a result of the functioning process is a question for debate. It certainly has an effect on the response to stimuli and the resulting adaptation process. Care must be taken to ensure that the aspect of self-concept is included in the assessment.

Use of this assessment approach requires a knowledge of systems theory and an understanding of the concepts and terminology related to adaptation theory. Some time may be required to orient the personnel involved in the activity before the assessment can begin. The audience for whom the assessment is intended should also be considered. Care should be taken to define pertinent vocabulary and key concepts. A common pitfall of health professionals is to become so attuned to their own jargon that they forget it may not be understandable to those outside the profession.

CONSIDERATIONS IN SELECTING AND EVALUATING DATA

Determining Initial Impressions

The assessment process entails a number of interrelated steps. Information is collected, interpreted, clustered, and a conclusion is drawn.

Observations lead to inferences which guide the observers in gathering additional data. As this cyclical process continues, connections are made among pieces of assessment data based on the knowledge of the person doing the assessment. This clustering of information is facilitated by a predetermined conceptual approach to assessment. This conceptual approach may be a mental status examination; a head-to-toe, or review of systems, format; an epidemiological investigation; or Kent's descriptive approach.

This process requires the use of clinical judgment. Gordon states that judgment "implies careful evaluation and assertion of an opinion based on specialized knowledge."[1] Therefore, not only is the degree of skillfulness in data collection influenced by clinical knowledge, but the interpretation of cues, or drawing inferences from data, requires clinical knowledge.

As students learn physical assessment skills, they readily develop the skill or technical dexterity required to perform the assessment technique. However, the clinical judgment required to interpret the data obtained does not develop so quickly. Similarly, the ability to determine what additional data should be gathered in order to clarify the meaning of certain signs or symptoms comes only with numerous experiences assessing a variety of clients. The following are some questions a nurse might ask in assessing an individual. What does a blood pressure of 170/90 mean? What else does the nurse need to know to interpret its meaning? Was this reading taken on an 85-year-old woman under treatment for hypertension or on a 14-year-old during a blood pressure screening program at school? A teacher refers a child to the school nurse because of a rash. The nurse must determine whether the child should be excluded from school, referred to a physician, or returned to class. What does the rash look like in color, structure, and location? Has the child been in contact with a communicable skin disorder or a food or a substance that could cause such a rash? Does the child have a history of previous skin disorders or allergies?

Some data are less complex to interpret, other data are more difficult. Often it requires the nurse to be knowledgeable in pathophysiology, developmental differences, risk factors, pharmacology, psychodynamics, and human behavior to determine the underlying causes for signs and symptoms or behavior initially assessed.

These processes of interpretation of the meaning of assessment data are just as applicable to community assessment as to an assessment of an individual. When a nurse walks through a community and observes fences around most of the homes, the nurse may wonder if this indicates a high value on privacy, a concern for security, a large proportion of families with dogs, or a norm established at a particular time when the houses were built. Other observations and interview data will help clarify the meaning of this one observation. Are neighbors visiting back and forth over these fences? Does everyone seem to know everyone, or do the people seem to feel, "I don't know my neighbors. Everyone keeps to his own business here"? Are they concerned about the crime rate in the neighborhood, and do the police department statistics support such a concern? The answers to each of these questions give direction for further assessment. It is important that a series of observations is made and perceptions are checked out with members of the community to assure accurate interpretation of observations.

Sampling

When a nurse assesses a client, it is not possible to know everything there is to know about that community, nor is it necessary. Many factors affect the kind and amount of assessment data collected. Most communities are too large to be able to observe or to interview everyone. The nurse must gather data from a portion or sample of the population and/or environment. Certainly the immediacy and severity of the presenting problem may force the nurse to greatly limit the focus of the sample of assessment data. This is true when an epidemic occurs that either has a high attack rate or is causing deaths or acute illness. Sufficient data must be collected to identify effective points interrupting the epidemic, and action must be taken even before a thorough understanding of the factors involved in its development can be determined. As indicated in the previous section, the sample must be large enough to assure accurate interpretation of data and that the data collected truly reflects what is happening in the community. Other factors that affect the focus of sampled data have been previously discussed in Chapter 2.

Multiple Sources of Data

The nurse quickly learns in assessing an individual that data from multiple sources are required before an accurate picture of the client is available from which a conclusion or nursing diagnosis may be drawn. Multiple sources require a variety of assessment techniques—history, interview regarding chief complaint, observation, and direct physical assessment techniques. They also require exploration of multiple body systems or multiple dimensions; that is, physical, cultural, psychological, sociological, and spiritual.

This is also true in assessing a community. Data from observations, interviews, census tract, knowledge of risk groups all combine to provide a picture of the community and its possible problems and needs. Therefore, the nurse cannot conclude from making an observation of many children playing in a low-income area that there is a need for an immunization clinic without further assessing immunization levels in the population, the use of existing resources, and the occurrence of communicable disease in the population.

Accuracy of Data

How well information is remembered and reported is one concern when determining the accuracy of data being collected. The sequence of events must be clearly described. This is a critical factor in assessing a food outbreak in a community.

Another factor to consider is the degree of trust developed between the persons providing the information and the nurse performing the assessment. Just as it is necessary to develop rapport with individual clients in order to obtain accurate responses, it is necessary that community members see the nurse as trustworthy.

Another aspect of the concept of trusting someone with information has to do with the investment a person has in the situation. In doing community assessments, one often finds that members of a community will be protective of their community and deny or diminish the problem. It is not unusual to see this behavior in individuals. Only after rapport has been developed and assessment data clarified does the problem become apparent. This is particularly true where there is a high potential for value judgments or legal implications; for instance, a problem of child abuse or drug dependency.

There may also be biases in sources of data selected for the assessment. If the community is diverse in age, ethnicity, or values, focusing the assessment on one segment of the population will bias the results. If a group of citizens are particularly concerned about an issue, they may provide biased information to the nurse assessing the community in which they reside. For instance, "old-time" residents in an apartment building in a downtown area that has traditionally housed low-income elderly but that recently has a growing number of young adult male residents may be very concerned about their safety without any particular incident to provide supporting assessment data. Biased data may be supplied intentionally or unintentionally. Biased data reflect a group's perception of the situation and values, and the nurse must take this into account in interpreting these data. Nevertheless, these data are real and have meaning for the individuals involved.

Another common concern in interpreting information is the fact that often the boundaries of the community the nurse is assessing may not match those for the area included in the assessment data available. For instance, the census tract or other geographical area from which published information is available may include many more people than those in the neighborhood that the nurse is assessing. Air pollution or air quality indicators often are reported for a whole city, yet the air quality may vary greatly among the downtown, industrial, or suburban residential areas.

Another aspect is the reliability of the data. Under different circumstances would the same piece of information mean the same thing? Some data are more reliable than other data. The previous example of interpreting the meaning of fences in a neighborhood led to a wide range of possible conclusions. Therefore, fencing is not as reliable a criterion for determining crime in a community as are the crime statistics developed by the police department.

Validity of Information

The question of validity of assessment data seems to revolve around the determination of the degree of relevance the information has in establishing a diagnosis. Gordon defines a valid cue as one that is "a critical defining characteristic" of the diagnosis.[2] Cues or signs and symptoms that are irrelevant in establishing one diagnosis may be indicators of another problem. Gordon states that "each piece of clinical data collected should provide additional information relevant to judgment about a functional health problem."[3] However, some degree of redundancy in cues is important to verify the impressions or interpretations made on existing data. The assessor looks for cues that are usually, frequently, or nearly always associated with a problem. When determining the cause of an outbreak of diarrhea, the investigator gathers information about signs and symptoms and the time frame for development of symptoms in order to differentiate between staphylococcal food poisoning and salmonella infection.

Some cues have a higher degree of accuracy in predicting a problem than others; those cues which have a more vague relationship with a problem are followed up by gathering information on more valid indicators. Cues that are quite relevant to an assessment are those which 1) signify change in the client's own personal pattern, 2) indicate deviation from the "norm," 3) indicate behavior that is nonproductive within the context of the whole client, and 4) indicate the development of a pattern that may be nonfunctional for the client.[4] For instance, a community experiences a series of rapes that is in excess to the number experienced in previous years. As a result of this experience, the previously open and friendly community becomes very distrustful of strangers. Numerous evening social activities are cancelled, and they are not reestablished even after the apprehension of the rapist. This example indicates a change in the community's pattern of behavior which may be nonproductive or nonfunctional for the community.

Clustering Information

With increasing expertise in assessment, the nurse learns to look for patterns within the data and to package the information in such a manner that commonalities are determined and signs and symptoms commonly occurring together are identified. These judgments form the data base supporting nursing diagnoses. This is what Kent refers to as themes in the Descriptive Approach to community assessment. In performing this task, it is important that the nurse not reject or discount significant data because they do not fit the nurse's predetermined conceptual package of data. Such variation from the expected should serve warning to investigate the meaning of those data. It is important to be very careful of biases or prejudices on the part of the assessor. Thus, it is imperative that data be clearly descriptive of the observation with no interpretation or judgment at this point.

Validating Assumptions

All these considerations in clinical judgment lead to the necessity of validating the assumptions the nurse makes during initial and ongoing data collection. According to Phipps,[5] inferences made on assessment data should be validated through comparison with an authoritative source, with concomitant data or cues, clarification with the client's perceptions, and/or obtaining verification from a reference group. An example of an authoritative source in community assessment would be air quality standards established by the Environmental Protection Agency. Comparing the observed value with the expected value requires the nurse to be knowledgeable in expected values. Concomitant data would include both the concept of determining whether or not data from subsequent assessments are consistent with previously collected data as well as determining if data from multiple sources using a variety of techniques confirm findings. For example, do data from the physical assessment, lab values, client history, and presenting complaints agree with each other? Do the observations of a community; review of mortality, morbidity, and demographic statistics; and survey of health concerns all lead to the same conclusions? It is important to clarify with clients their perceptions of the meaning of observed data. If you are in a semirural community where the homes are surrounded by a large amount of farm equipment in various stages of repair, is this seen as an "eyesore" or environmental hazard, or is it a status symbol or at least a norm with that community? Nurses often are part of a team involved in performing a community assessment. Members of the team may serve as a reference group in which each member may "check out" interpretations of data with the other team members.

As previously indicated, observations lead to inferences which lead to further observations which either confirm or question initial impressions. This process continues until sufficient data are available to formulate a tentative diagnosis

REFERENCES

1. GORDON, M: *Nursing Diagnosis: Process and Application.* McGraw-Hill, New York, 1982, p 14.
2. Ibid, p 134.
3. Ibid, p 128.
4. Ibid, p 137.
5. PHIPPS, W, LONG, B, WOOD, NF: *Medical-Surgical Nursing.* CV Mosby, St Louis, 1979, pp 92–93.

CHAPTER 9

COMMUNITY DIAGNOSIS

OBJECTIVES

THE LEARNER WILL

1. define the term community diagnosis.

2. formulate a diagnostic statement when given sample assessment data.

3. arrange community diagnoses in an organized format.

4. discuss the implications of community assessment activities for nursing practice.

Conclusions or judgments about the data collected are developed as a natural outcome of the assessment process. Conclusions give labels or names to the problem situations. These names are known as diagnoses. Diagnoses are hypotheses regarding health problems, concerns, and health achievements.

They are sometimes considered a part of the assessment phase of the problem-solving process or may be designated a separate step between assessment and planning.[1] Just as hypotheses in research give definition to the situation as viewed by the researcher, the diagnosis identifies the condition of the client from the perspective of the health professional.

It is only fairly recently that the term "diagnosis" has been used in fields other than medicine, even though all health professionals who participate in assisting clients with the resolution of health problems are involved in developing diagnoses. Each profession directs its diagnostic statements toward the activities that are its area of expertise. Medicine is involved with the diagnosis and treatment of disease. Social work is concerned with the psychological, psychiatric, economic, and social aspects of the population. The arena for nursing is the *potential or actual "functional coping deficits" of a client.*[2]

Concentrating on the diagnosis of potential or actual functional problems using nursing diagnoses is appropriate when the community is viewed as a client with the ability or inability to function in order to meet its own needs. This broadens the focus to include response to disease, social problems, or any area in which the community client needs assistance in order to function effectively. The term "community diagnosis" is used to differentiate diagnoses related to the community client from diagnoses related to individuals or families within a community or individuals influenced by a community.[3] Although the diagnosis is based on activities related to nursing, using the designation community diagnosis also gives recognition to the common practice of an interdisciplinary approach to community health problems.

Nursing has made a deliberate effort to define the concept of nursing diagnosis and to develop a diagnostic language and classification related to health problems that deal with functional deficits. Although attention has been directed primarily to the individual, the language and classification system can be adapted to the formulation of community diagnoses.

DIAGNOSTIC STATEMENT

Once the assessment data have been accumulated and organized, a clear statement of the problem must be formulated. This statement will serve as the basis for further action in the problem-solving process. It must accurately depict the situation as made evident by the information available and must be expressed in a language that is understandable. This statement is the diagnosis.

The diagnostic statement consists of two segments. The first part identifies the problem such as "lack of understanding," "anxiety," or "nutrition." Usually there are some modifying words attached to clarify or to define better the magnitude of the problem like "potential lack of understanding," "acute anxiety," or "increasing nutritional deficits."

The intent for formulating a diagnosis is not only to state conclusions but also to provide guidance for planning. Generalized words such as "acute anxiety" express conclusions regarding the client which identify the problem area and its severity. Further description is necessary in order to give direction for assisting the client to cope with the problem. The second part of the statement provides this clarification by giving information describing the circumstances or reasons for the problem occurrence. This part is usually connected to the first with the transitional words "due to," "related to," or "secondary to." A complete diagnostic statement for a community might be "acute anxiety related to the abduction of two children from the area."

A diagnosis, like a hypothesis, is tentative. It is based on current objective data and subject to revision as new information is presented. The act of formulating a diagnosis puts conclusions and judgments into a concrete expression which gives direction for management of health care.

There may be several statements addressing a number of specific problem areas. It is also possible to identify the general problem with a diagnostic statement and to develop *subdiagnoses* which would assist the client in coping with the primary functional deficit. A nurse who does this is like a teacher who might identify a broad, general learning objective with several specific subobjectives to give direction for reaching the general objective.

Carnevalli[4] suggests that these more specific subdiagnoses be termed the *working diagnoses*. These working diagnoses result in individualized care appropriate to that particular problem situation. For the previous example, "acute anxiety related to the abduction of two children from the area," some working diagnoses might be

1. Moderate anxiety related to the safety of children walking to and from school.
2. Lack of understanding of normal police procedure related to the abduction of a child.
3. Grieving caused by the loss of two children from the neighborhood.

ORGANIZATION OF DIAGNOSES

The National Conferences for Classification of Nursing Diagnoses have directed their efforts since 1973 toward a standardization of nursing diagnoses by developing diagnoses which can be accepted by the nursing profession.[5] This effort has centered primarily on the individual and is moving toward consideration of family concerns and problems. Simmons[6] has developed a classification scheme for client problems to be used in community health nursing for the U.S. Department of Health and Human Services. Here, again, attention is focused on the individual members of the community population rather than on the community as a client.

Gordon[7] has taken another step in the development of the process by grouping nursing diagnoses into categories she terms "functional health patterns." This categorization also represents the initiation of a standardized assessment format. The patterns include

1. Health-Perception—Health-Management
2. Nutritional—Metabolic
3. Elimination
4. Activity—Exercise
5. Cognitive—Perceptual
6. Sleep—Rest
7. Self-perception—Self-concept
8. Role—Relationship
9. Sexuality—Reproduction
10. Coping—Stress tolerance
11. Value—Belief.[8]

The functional health patterns assessment format identifies areas of assessment for the community client within each category, as well as for the individual and family, using the currently accepted diagnostic key words from the Conferences on Nursing Diagnoses. Gordon very carefully established her assessment categories so that they were unaffected by the approach used by the health professional collecting the data. They simply allow the collected information to be grouped in a standardized way and promote a comprehensive assessment.

This process of organizing diagnoses which started with an emphasis on the individual client can produce results that are sometimes awkward and unclear when they are applied to the community client. It is impossible, for example, to translate an assessment of sleep-rest patterns of the community to mean an assessment of increased levels of stress because of sleep-rest disturbances, as Gordon has done. Stress then becomes the assessment category, with sleep-rest disturbances the cause. This can also be interpreted as an illustration of an assessment of individuals within the community rather than of the community client.

In an effort to accomplish the same objective, Andrews[9] uses theoretical models based on structure and process as guides for the development of community diagnoses. Each model generates its own particular type of diagnoses. An assessment using demographic characteristics as the model might direct the investigator to assess health problems such as infant mortality or chronic disease. A systems model base tends toward consideration of relationships within the community and with its environment. This approach for identifying diagnoses would give direction to the formulation of the diagnoses and would give consideration to the community as the client, but the lack of a standardized format might lead to some gaps in identification of problem areas. The theoretical models vary in their emphasis because some are based on structure and others on process.

The idea of some universal categories for organizing community assessment data, no matter which conceptual approach is utilized in the assessment process, is important. Because community diagnoses describe functional deficits, another way of categorizing them might be in relation to the previously identified functions of a community:

1. Utilization of space—housing, access and egress, socialization, and recreation.

2. Means of livelihood—employment, sustenance, health
3. Production, distribution, consumption of goods and services
4. Protection of its members—creating and enforcing norms and controls, prevention of physical disasters
5. Education—socialization of adults, children and newcomers, ongoing enrichment
6. Participation—communication, social interaction, support
7. Linkage with other systems providing for needs of its members when the community is unable or elects not to carry out its function.

The items listed in the functional health patterns used by Gordon and the community health concerns based on theoretical models proposed by Andrews fit into this system of categorization. It also serves to support the concept of the community as the direct client. The following example illustrates how nursing diagnostic statements and a category system based on community functions listed above can be used in developing community diagnoses.

A Community in Crisis

The community of Spokane, Washington, experienced a natural disaster when Mount St. Helens erupted in May of 1980. A giant cloud of volcanic ash was blown by air currents in an easterly direction. Large amounts of ash fell to the ground as the cloud moved along. By noon the town of Moses Lake, Washington, began to feel the effects of the eruption, and around 3 PM in Spokane the cloud obscured the sunlight so that the street lights came on and the ash was falling everywhere.

There were no warnings or announcements on any of the radio and television stations between the time of the eruption and 3 o'clock. The emergency broadcasting system did not function until the cloud had enveloped the city. A great crowd of people had driven to nearby Fairchild Air Force Base to attend an air show and found themselves forced to return, somehow, through the darkness and encompassing gray ash.

The event was unexpected as far as the general population was concerned. No one had any previous experience with volcanic ash. There was a general feeling of alarm, anxiety, fear, and for some an excitement and exhilaration in experiencing something new and unusual. The calming effect produced by participating in some part of preparatory activities had not occurred.

Listed below are some of the major functional areas of a community and some concerns and reactions of the population during this disaster:

1. *Shelter.* People were stranded in cars, the airport, hotels, motels, and homes. Those in transit were housed at the emergency station at one of the local high schools.
2. *Transportation.* Movement of cars, buses, trains, and airplanes was halted within Spokane and between Spokane and the rest of the coun-

try. There was a ban on all driving, and no one was sure of the effects of the ash to automobile engines.

3. *Food.* Some people did not have adequate food supplies in their homes. At first most restaurants and grocery stores were closed. During the ban on traffic, emergency services were used to bring food to people unable to obtain it. As the stores began to open, there was a "run" on certain commodities in stores. Some people hoarded food. Neighbors borrowed and shared food supplies. Others walked to obtain food for those less mobile.

4. *Water.* There was a concern about possible water contamination. Some people filled their bathtub with water and put bottles of water aside in case something happened to the water or the power.

5. *Electricity.* It was unknown whether the ash would affect the power supply system in some way.

6. *Air.* This was the major area of anxiety. People were worried about possible damage from the ash to their lungs and eyes, car or house paint, pets and farm animals, yard, flowers, trees, property. Face masks were recommended for all who ventured outside. Stores ran out of supplies of masks. Eventually emergency supplies of masks could be obtained at local fire stations. There was much discussion about short- and long-range effects of inhaling the ash. Air filters for popular makes of cars were in short supply.

7. *Waste Disposal.* Disposition of the ash itself was a problem. Sweeping caused it to blow around and settle somewhere else. Emphasis was placed on community efforts to help the city clean the streets and sidewalks. Neighbors cooperated in hosing the accumulation into the storm drains along with the assistance of firehoses. Spokane had not upgraded its sewer system to include separate storm drains. It was unknown whether the ash would clog the sewer system somehow and what its effects would be on the rivers and fish. Heavy use of water for the cleaning activities reduced water pressure in some neighborhoods.

8. *Health.* Short-range concerns were irritation to air passages and eyes. Long-range concerns were the uncertainties of the effects of the ash to the human body. Other immediate concerns were of those with chronic lung conditions, those who needed new supplies of medications, and those who needed medical or nursing services.

9. *Sense of Well Being.* Some of the people were anxious and uneasy. They were concerned about what to do or not to do, could not focus and use time effectively, were worried about the outcome of the situation for themselves and significant others. Some felt at a loss because of the interruption of routines and normal roles. Others enjoyed the change, stimulation of a new challenge, and an opportunity to share the situation with their neighbors.

10. *Economy.* All businesses were closed for almost a week. There were a loss of commerce during that time, a loss of work time, and the cost of clean up. A major part of Spokane's economy is based on agriculture.

The questionable impact of the ash on the current year's crops as well as the future effects were unknown.

11. *Governance.* A state of emergency was declared, and the following directions were given to the public: There was to be no driving. People were to stay home. No businesses or schools would be open. In case of an emergency, speed-limit restrictions would be enforced and there would be ticketing for nonemergency travel.

   Road blocks and closing of highways occurred. The use of police power was limited. In some areas the National Guard was used to help clean up. Alternate day water usage was requested to wash off houses and clean streets. Possible citations could be issued for not cleaning up.

12. *Institutions.* Schools and colleges were closed. Churches and other organizations cancelled regular meetings. Post offices were closed. Governmental business, except for that related to the emergency, came to a standstill.

13. *Communication.* As soon as the disaster occurred, the Emergency Broadcasting System and local radio stations kept the public constantly informed of the latest information. Making and receiving telephone calls were difficult the first few days. Mail was disrupted. It was difficult to reach significant others in the affected areas or for those within the area to let others know they were doing well.

14. *Socialization/Recreational Activities.* Outdoor activities were discontinued; the YMCA, theaters, restaurants, and bars were closed. Schools, organizations, and work settings which provide socialization were also closed. In some cases neighborhood interaction increased during the clean-up or individuals and groups within a neighborhood found innovative ways to socialize within the confines of the emergency restrictions.

15. *Community Spirit.* There was no panic, and there were many volunteers. Homeowners and businesses did what was asked of them. They almost overwhelmed the water system while hosing down the streets. Emergency services such as the Red Cross, fire department, and police department were used. Amtrak ran a free train-lift through the affected area to transport those stranded to ash-free Seattle. People felt an increased sense of identity with the community and its residents.

The resulting concerns or problems can be arranged into groups according to the functions of a community. A disaster of this magnitude would, of course, generate numerous diagnoses. For the purposes of this example, a single community diagnosis is proposed for each category to serve as an illustration of the possibilities for planning.

COMMUNITY FUNCTION	COMMUNITY DIAGNOSIS
Utilization of space	Alteration in self-care ability of community members related to need for tempo-

	rary shelter and travel restrictions.
Means of livelihood	Impaired community management related to business closure.
Goods and services	Potential economic coping deficit related to disruption of business and agricultural activities.
Protection	Possible noncompliance with emergency rules and regulations related to lack of communication.
Education/Socialization	Lack of knowledge of the effects of the ash owing to the uniqueness of the situation.
Participation	Impaired communication and social interaction related to physical isolation.
Linkage with other systems	Potential ineffective community coping related to inability to bear the total cost of clean-up endeavors.

IMPLICATIONS FOR NURSING PRACTICE

Once the community diagnoses have been established, the assessment phase of the nursing process is concluded. The planning phase then begins with the determination of priorities. At this point the nurse will need to determine the degree to which the problems are within the scope of nursing practice. The problems may be addressed directly from a nursing perspective, may require cooperative endeavors among health providers, or may be primarily outside the scope of nursing practice and require referral.

Regardless of whether the nurse has been the primary person performing the assessment or a member of a team, the problems identified frequently require an interdisciplinary effort to assist the community to meet the expressed needs. The nurse must know or be able to identify individuals with relevant expertise with whom to plan programs jointly. The individuals may be within the formal or informal political arena, the business sector of the community, the health care provider sector, or the sector of the community that will become the primary consumer of the program's services.

It is important that the nurse jointly plan with these groups rather than identify problems and abdicate responsibility for participating in planning for their solutions. Taking the latter approach often results in no movement toward solutions because those able to make the changes may not have developed the commitment to do so. Even when the need(s) that have highest priority must be met by a program that does not require direct delivery of nursing service, these programs have an impact on the well-being of the community as an entity. The nurse plays a critical role in monitoring the health implications of such projects. Nursing and health services frequently are delivered within the context of a larger project, and it is vitally important that nurses influence the plans for projects which will have impact on delivery of health care.

Depending upon the organizational structure of the agency within which the nurse functions, the staff nurse may directly participate in these endeavors or the supervisor may be more involved in interdisciplinary planning with consultation from the nurse or nurses involved in the original assessment. There are numerous instances in rural areas, schools, and industries in which the staff may consist of one, two, or at most three nurses. The staff level nurse must be able to directly initiate and participate in the program-planning process.

The needs identified from the assessment data may be directly met by development of nursing programs, for example, exercise or stress reduction class, health screening for identified high-risk groups, or hospice services. The nurse may need to work with relevant community groups and agencies to plan for such problems. Or priorities within the nurse's practice may be reordered to allow the nurse to develop and to initiate the program.

A community assessment may indicate gaps in available information crucial to planning which require further assessment before the planning process may begin. The assessment may have served the role of a preliminary study in research; that is, an initial exploration of an area of concern which provides the information necessary to design a research study. Even when the focus is upon development of services to meet identified needs, the planning of such programs should include the development of criteria and methodology by which the program outcomes will be evaluated. This process is known as evaluation research.

Just as the nurse's goal is to encourage as much independence as possible within individual and family clients, the nurse working with a community should encourage and assist the community to solve its own health problems. Regardless of the approach to planning and whether the complexity of the problem and the nurse's degree of expertise suggest the nurse is the leader or member of the planning endeavor, the nurse will need to be able to 1) organize and present assessment data in such a manner that they clearly support the conclusions drawn (community diagnoses), 2) sell the necessity to plan for meeting the identified needs, and 3) assist in development of a plan to meet these needs, which includes allocation or acquisition of additional resources or reallocation of existing resources either within the agency or from other sources within or outside the community.

REFERENCES

1. BOWER, FL: *The Process of Planning Nursing Care*, ed 3. CV Mosby, St Louis, 1982, p 17.

2. WALTER, J, PARDEE, G, MOLBO, D: *Dynamics of Problem-Oriented Approaches: Patient Care and Documentation*. JB Lippincott, Philadelphia, 1976, p 53.

3. HAMILTON, P: *Community nursing diagnoses.* ANS, April 1983, pp 21–36.
4. CARNEVALLI, DL: *Nursing Care Planning: Diagnosis and Management.* JB Lippincott, Philadelphia, 1983.
5. KIM, MJ, MORITZ, DA: *Classification of Nursing Diagnosis.* McGraw-Hill, New York, 1982, pp 281–282.
6. SIMMONS, D: *A Classification Scheme for Client Problems in Community Health Nursing.* US Department of Health and Human Services, Hyattsville, MD, June 1980.
7. GORDON, M: *Nursing Diagnosis: Process and Application.* McGraw-Hill, New York, 1982, Appendix B, pp 327–328.
8. Ibid, pp 81–108.
9. ANDREWS, PB: *Nursing diagnosis.* In GRIFFITH, J AND CHRISTENSEN, P: *Nursing Process: Application and Theories, Frameworks and Models.* CV Mosby, St Louis, 1982.

UNIT BIBLIOGRAPHY

ANDREWS, PB: *Nursing diagnosis.* In GRIFFITH, J AND CHRISTENSEN, P: *Nursing Process: Application and Theories, Frameworks and Models.* CV Mosby, St Louis, 1982.

BOWER, FL: *The Process of Planning Nursing Care,* ed 3. CV Mosby, St. Louis, 1982.

CARNEVALLI, DL: *Nursing Care Planning: Diagnosis and Management.* JB Lippincott, Philadelphia, 1983.

ERICKSON, H, TOMLIN, E, SWAIN, MA: *Modeling and Role-Modeling.* Prentice-Hall, Englewood Cliffs, NJ, 1983.

GORDON, M: *Nursing Diagnosis: Process and Application.* McGraw-Hill, New York, 1982.

HAMILTON, P: *Community nursing diagnoses.* ANS, April 1983.

KIM, MJ AND MORITZ, DA: *Classification of Nursing Diagnosis.* McGraw-Hill, New York, 1982.

PHIPPS, W, LONG, B, WOOD, NF: *Medical-Surgical Nursing.* CV Mosby, St Louis, 1979.

SIMMONS, D: *A Classification Schedule for Client Problems in Community Health Nursing.* US Department of Health and Human Services, Hyattsville, MD, June 1980.

WALTER, J, PARDEE, G, MOLBO, D: *Dynamics of Problem-Oriented Approaches: Patient Care and Documentation.* JB Lippincott, Philadelphia, 1976.

CASE STUDIES IN COMMUNITY ASSESSMENT

Community assessment is all very well and good, you say, but how does it work in the real situation? Are the approaches useful? Would an investment in such an activity produce beneficial results? The following case studies are presented for contemplation and discussion. They illustrate a variety of experiences with community assessment. The examples have been chosen to demonstrate the applicability of community assessment in selected settings in which the professional nurse deals with the community as a client. They range from the retrospective account of a recent nursing graduate beginning a community health nursing experience to the use of community assessment as a teaching tool and learning exercise in a baccalaureate nursing program. It is hoped they will stimulate ideas and thoughts about the assessment phase of the nursing process in relation to the community client.

Grateful appreciation and acknowledgement is extended to the following creative and enthusiastic contributors: Tina Bayne, Jo McNeil, Katherine Chavigny, Linda Felver, and Donna Haw.

CHAPTER 10

A SUMMER CAMP COMMUNITY

TINA BAYNE, R.N., M.S.

Have you ever thought about a children's summer camp as a small, defined community needing assessment by the nurse? I didn't consider that possibility until my first job as a camp nurse. The situation described in this chapter is based upon my actual experiences as a new baccalaureate-prepared nurse at a summer camp.

St John's Landing Camp is a summer camp located within a state park in the Midwest. The camp covers about 2 square miles in a beautiful, rustic setting. A "wild river" forms one of the camp's natural boundaries (Fig. 10–1).

The camp consists of many pre-World War II type buildings. Major camp buildings are a mess hall/activities center, an arts and crafts shop, an administration building, an infirmary, and cabins for campers located in four different units, or areas, of the camp. The units are separated from each other by about one-half mile. Only a few camp buildings have electricity: the administration building, the mess hall/activities center, and the infirmary. Kerosene lanterns are used for lighting in the other areas.

St John's Landing Camp setting is lush with huge pine trees, wildflowers, and wildlife. It is not all that unusual to "bump" into a deer when walking along an unlit path at night. There are no concrete pathways within the camp. Nature has been left at its best.

The "community" of St John's Landing Camp consists of campers, counselors, and support staff. About 100 to 120 campers attend the camp for one of four 12-day sessions during the June–August camp season. The campers are boys and girls ages 9 through 13 from a nearby large metropolitan area. Many have

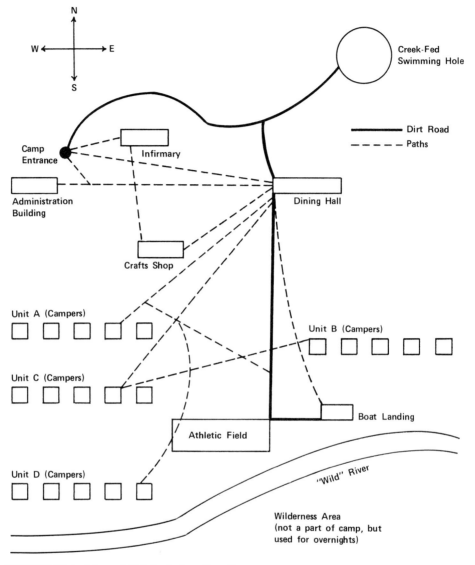

FIGURE 10-1. Map of St John's Landing Camp.

attended St John's Landing Camp in previous summers. The campers are delightful, energetic children.

St John's Landing Camp has a counselor and support staff of 24. The camp director, who is a school administrator, is the direct supervisor of the camp. Three cooks are hired from the local area. Most of the other staff are college students. There are 14 counselors, two unit directors, two waterfront directors, an arts and crafts director, and the camp nurse. I entered this community some years ago as St John's Landing Camp's camp nurse, a challenging position which I held for two summers.

ROLE OF THE NURSE

My role as camp nurse at St John's Landing Camp was loosely defined. I had a one-page job description that listed a number of mandatory duties that the camp nurse must do: review health history forms, administer medications as necessary to campers, provide first aid services, and so forth. I quickly realized that it was up to me to further define my role based on the health needs of this small defined community. My primary goal was to make the camp a healthy place for campers, counselors, and staff.

I began by investigating what the camp nurse had done in previous summers. Unfortunately, no records could be found from the last nurse. The camp director, my immediate supervisor, was supportive but had little recall of "specifics." He gave only vague answers to my questions about the frequency and types of camp accidents, the usual number of 35-mile trips to the local emergency room, and the times of day previously designated by the nurse for "sick call." I also had been hoping for a note from last summer's nurse expressing some of the joys and frustrations of the job. I mentally made a note that I would leave such a letter for the camp nurse who would follow me at St John's Landing Camp.

I learned a great deal about the camp from the counselors and other staff and from my observations of what was going on at the camp. I taught first aid and cardiopulmonary resuscitation review classes for the staff. I established a working relationship with the local physician. Quickly I developed accident protocols and an accident-prevention program. I didn't realize it then, but in attempting to gain a historical perspective and in conducting my interviews with "key" people I had begun my community assessment. That assessment would provide the basis for the development of my camp nurse role over the summer.

As St John's Landing Camp's nurse, I found it helpful to look at the camp as a whole—in a way, to stand back and to see what was really happening within the camp. In gaining this broader view, I was able to identify potential problems with the camp environment and help reformulate some of the procedures and policies of the camp. Exciting things began to happen as my "camp nurse" interventions were started. The following cases are examples of interventions based on assessment of the community.

Case Situation A

Within the first few days of camp, I began to notice that I was seeing between five and ten campers daily with foot injuries and foot conditions, for example, cuts, scrapes, and infections. I also noticed that many of the campers, and some of the counselors, walked barefoot throughout the camp a fair portion of the time. I talked with the unit directors and some of the counselors and found that foot injuries were always a common occurrence. There never had been a camp policy about the wearing of shoes. So one of my first interventions was to establish a camp rule that shoes were to be worn at all times, except at the swimming areas.

After initiation of the rule, the number of campers with foot injuries decreased dramatically. One new problem arose: a few of the children came to camp with badly worn shoes, which disintegrated within the first few days at camp. This problem, however, was handled by the camp's purchase of several pairs of thongs and tennis shoes.

Case Situation B

"We swim every day at SJLC." That phrase was frequently stated by the camp's two waterfront directors. Half the campers swim every morning, and the other half, every afternoon. The camp's major swimming area is a creek-fed "swimming hole" approximately one half mile down a sandy camp road (See Figure 10–1.).

One of my major fears was a drowning accident. I observed that everyone walked to and from the swimming area each day. I noted that in the event of a potential drowning or other serious accident at the swimming area there would be no way to quickly transport the injured individual back to the main camp area for treatment by the camp nurse and/or possible transfer to the local emergency room. No one had explored the need for emergency transportation, inasmuch as there had never been a serious accident at the swimming area. A nursing intervention seemed essential, however, to reduce the time that might be lost transporting an injured individual. The solution proved to be very simple. I suggested that the waterfront directors drive a car to the swimming area each day. The car could be used, if needed, for emergency transport. The suggestion was accepted as a camp policy—certainly a move in the direction of prevention!

Case Situation C

One of the directives I received from my camp director was that each camper was to be weighed and measured on entry to camp and on exit from camp. Essentially that meant that all campers were to be seen by me on day 1 and day 11. The weighing and measuring process was a tedious one, especially with the antiquated scale at camp. The process also consumed a fair portion of time for me and the campers.

After the first session of camp, I questioned the camp director as to the purpose of the measurements. He had no idea of why they should be done, other than that the camp health form provided a blank for the height and weight information. He seemed reluctant to abolish the procedure.

I continued the same process for one more session but found that the results of the weighing and measuring were useless. The children weren't at camp long enough to make a significant difference in their measurements. Also, I was convinced that the time I spent as a camp nurse in this activity could be better utilized. I wanted to meet with each group of campers, explain my role to them, and do some health teaching.

At the beginning of the third session of camp, I initiated a new procedure, with approval of the camp director. I met with each cabin group on the first day at camp on their way to swimming. I was able to briefly assess their skin and identify those campers who had brought medications or had other health concerns to share with me. I briefly introduced the campers to my role and to some of the camp rules, and I taught about safety. I also offered to weigh and measure campers who requested this service. This new approach worked well. Feedback from the counselors and campers was positive.

Case Situation D

Several weeks into the camp season I began to see several counselors and staff members in my office each day complaining of fatigue and colds. At one point, at least half the camp counselors and staff were sick. Something had to be done beyond cough medicine, rest, and fluids.

In looking at the camp environment, I noted lots of complaints about the food from the camp counselors and staff. The quality of food was not a problem, but the quantity was. Because of a tight budget, all people at camp received about the same amount of food at each meal. However, the nutritional needs of the 22-year-old counselor are not the same as the 10-year-old camper!

After some negotiations with the camp director and the cooks, I was able to arrange for nutritious snacks in adequate amounts for the counselors and staff each evening. This intervention was well received, and the counselors and staff made good use of the extra cheese, eggs, fruit, bread, peanut butter, and milk. It is interesting that after about a week the number of counselors and staff at "sick call" decreased. Although the improved diet cannot be given full credit for the improvement in health status, I do think it had an impact on the outcome.

Case Situation E

Sometime about halfway through the camp season, I started to see an increased number of campers with eye infections. I also noted that some of the campers had a similar mild generalized erythematous body rash. The histories elicited from these campers were essentially negative for anything out of the ordinary. The one thing in common was that all the campers went swimming daily at the swimminghole.

It seemed important to track down the possible cause for the increased number of campers with eye infections and body rashes. The swimminghole seemed the logical place to start. The swimming directors stated that the water in the swimminghole seemed to be more stagnant and murky than earlier in the summer. I contacted the park director and requested that the water in the swimminghole be tested for bacteria and other organisms. Results of the test indicated a need to change the water. The swimminghole was drained, cleaned, and refilled. After this procedure the incidence of campers with body rashes and eye infections decreased.

Conclusions

Three factors—time, availability, and ease of use—were important in my choice of assessment techniques for use at camp. Time was short: I only had four 12-day camp sessions. Therefore, the approaches to be used for assessment needed to be readily available. Ease of use was also a major concern. As camp nurse I was "on call" 24 hours a day. I didn't have the time or energy to formally carry out an extensive community assessment and then determine interventions. These steps went on almost simultaneously. As demonstrated in the case situations, the techniques I found to be most successful in my assessment were observations, key informant interviews, and environmental indices. To a less extent the epidemiological method, resource analysis, and the historical perspective technique were used. It would have been helpful had I been able to make more use of demographic data analysis, surveys, and other community assessment techniques; however, often the data needed were not available to me.

I found community assessment to be an extremely valuable tool at camp. I truly believe that I gained credibility because of my nursing interventions, based on my assessment of the camp community. As the summer progressed, it was exciting to see improvement in the health status of the camp population in specific areas. Certainly the potential risks to the population had decreased, and there was a heightened awareness of health, wellness, and accident prevention.

My role changed too. I was seen as a key person at St John's Landing Camp—a health counselor, a health teacher, and a health provider, as well as a member of the management team helping determine the overall and day-to-day functioning of the camp. It is important that the nurse assess the decision-making process, be incorporated into the organization, and be viewed as a valued member of the team. The development of a healthy camp environment became a primary responsibility for everyone at St John's Landing Camp.

RECOMMENDATIONS

Community assessment is useful for the nurse working in a summer camp. It would be helpful for the nurse to begin gathering assessment information immediately. I think it is particularly helpful to talk with or to have information from the previous camp nurse. Counselors and other staff members who have been at camp before are also knowledgeable and should be consulted. The nurse needs to initiate interventions based on an assessment of the camp environment as well as the camp's procedures and policies. Improvement of the health status of the camp community, as a whole, needs to be the primary concern. When the techniques of community assessment are used, camp nursing can be a rewarding, fun experience!

CHAPTER 11

A PREGNANT SCHOOL-AGE COMMUNITY

TINA BAYNE, R.N., M.S.

The school-age population, although most often healthy, is at risk for a variety of health-related problems. The nurse working with students is in a unique position to assess the health status of individuals, groups of students, and the student population as a whole and to deliver health services to this distinct population.

Jones School is a small public school in a large metropolitan city. The school houses the city's special education program for pregnant junior and senior high school students.

The situation described in this chapter is based upon my experience as a public health/school nurse at Jones School. The local health district funded my position through a special projects grant for maternity and infant care. The grant provided for a full-time public health nurse to serve as the school nurse at Jones.

The emphasis of this chapter is on my assessment of the pregnant adolescent community as a whole and on the interventions I initiated based on my assessment of the student community at Jones.

I found community assessment to be a valuable tool. Although I did not do a systematic, extensive assessment of this pregnant adolescent community, I did employ the techniques of observations, resource analysis, key informant interviews, and environmental indices in my assessment of this community. I also found the epidemiological method, the historical perspective technique, and demographic data analysis to be useful. I found it critical to engage in ongoing assessment of the community because looking at a community at only one point in time severely limits the accuracy of the assessment.

CHARACTERISTICS OF THE COMMUNITY

Each community has unique characteristics which distinguish it from any other. This pregnant adolescent community indeed was a special population with numerous distinctive qualities. In the city described, adolescent students may choose to remain at their home school or transfer to Jones School during their pregnancy. Jones School has special services available to students. In addition to seven faculty, office personnel, and a school director, Jones School employs a full-time school social worker and a part-time counselor.

Jones School offers all the required academic subjects, as well as some electives. An infant care course is required for all students. The school program follows the academic year from September to June. The school day runs from 9 AM to 2:00 PM, Monday through Friday. The students travel to and from school via city buses or private transportation.

Between 60 and 100 students are enrolled at Jones at different times during the school year. Statistics show that approximately one half the city's pregnant teenagers choose to attend Jones School. Students at Jones range in age from 12 to 19 years. A student may elect to enroll in Jones School at any time during her pregnancy. Homebound tutoring is available for the student immediately after delivery until she is able to return to school. After delivery, most students return to their home school.

There are other features unique to Jones. As each girl registers in the program, she is interviewed by three people. First, the school counselor meets the girl and makes an initial assessment of her present school status. This includes past attendance record, scholastic record, and school behavior problems. Second, the girl sees the social worker, who makes an initial social assessment. This includes discussion of current and past relationships of the girl with her family and husband or boyfriend, assessment of financial need, and, in many instances, discussion of referral to a social agency that can follow the girl on an ongoing basis throughout her pregnancy. The social worker also explains to the student what she might anticipate at Jones, particularly the changes from her former school. The school nurse at Jones is the third person to interview students at admission.

ROLE OF THE SCHOOL NURSE

My role as school nurse was well defined by my public health nurse (PHN) supervisor, a maternal-child health specialist. She provided me with clear guidelines, frequent feedback, and a great deal of support throughout the school year. A few of my activities at Jones are described below.

I met with each student for an initial assessment interview upon her entry to school. I asked the student questions about her past and present health history and her source of prenatal care. When a student had no current source of health care, I attempted to help her find an appropriate medical source. I acquainted the student with my role at school and let her know that I was available to answer her health and pregnancy-related questions.

During the first interview, I also laid the foundation for a PHN referral to the local health department. A PHN was often able to provide one-to-one home visits throughout the student's pregnancy and postpartum period. I found that the PHNs provided invaluable support and health teaching to the students. I communicated with these nurses frequently.

At Jones, I was available to meet the individual needs of students by taking blood pressure, weighing a student, or discussing a particular health concern. Because of the small enrollment, I grew to know each of the students by name. It was a rewarding experience for me to get to know the students so well.

The school nurse's office at Jones School is a large comfortable classroom. There is plenty of bulletin board space for information on nutrition, exercise, infant development, and pregnancy. A variety of health-related pamphlets are available for students. The room also has a scale, so I encouraged students to "weigh in" frequently and to follow the growth of their fetus during pregnancy by using a prenatal weight gain grid.

All students at Jones were involved in "Nurse's Group," held 1 hour weekly for 10 weeks. Each group was made up of no more than 10 students sharing similar estimated days of confinement. A few of the topics covered at the nurse's group were nutrition, physical and psychological changes of pregnancy, labor, delivery, and birth control. The group was held in the large comfortable classroom described above.

Health at Jones did not begin or end with the school nurse. The faculty and staff attempted to establish an atmosphere conducive to the biological, psychological, cultural, and sociological well being of the students. I often met informally with the social worker or school director. The counselor, social worker, nurse, director, and teachers met weekly to combine their assessments of individual students and to determine an ongoing plan of action regarding each student. The student's educational, social, and health needs were taken into consideration. Our aim was the total well being of our students.

The following cases are examples of interventions based on my assessment of the adolescent community at Jones. I found it essential to consider the student community as a whole and to integrate my activities with those of other faculty and staff when planning these interventions.

Situation A: Low-Birth-Weight Babies

Teenagers frequently give birth to low-birth-weight babies. With that in mind, I told each student at Jones that I was available to weigh them and to plot their prenatal weight gain on a prenatal weight gain grid at their convenience. After several months and the frequent weighing of many students, I found that most of the students were having slow weight gains—almost always their weight gains were below the "normal curve" on the form I used. I questioned the students

---

individually and in my classes about their eating habits. Lunch was not a problem. A hot, nutritious meal was available each day.

I further questioned the students about their breakfast and dinner habits. Although most students reported that they ate an evening meal, *most* stated that they *rarely* ate a nutritious breakfast. In fact, many students stated that they did not eat any breakfast. I took my concerns about this issue to the faculty and staff at a weekly staff meeting. Considering the population and limited period of contact with individual students, a breakfast program was proposed. The staff supported my suggestion of initiating a program such as this at Jones. The school director took our request for a school breakfast program to her supervisors. Within a short time every student at Jones was provided with cold cereal, milk, juice and toast each school day.

The students were pleased by the breakfast program, and nearly every student ate breakfast at school each day. It is interesting to note that our statistics showed that our students had a lower incidence of low-birth-weight babies (5 lbs 8 oz or less) that year than the population served by the city health department's maternity clinics. Although these populations are not identical, they are frequently compared because of the similar demographic characteristics.

Situation B: Exercise Class

At Jones, I assisted with the teaching of an exercise class for the students needing a physical education credit or desiring monitored exercise. One day while I was conducting the exercise class, one of the students right next to me had a grand mal seizure. The reaction I saw from the other students was predictable—terror, horror; few had ever seen a person have a seizure.

After I got the student safely to the floor, placed her on her side, and helped clear her airway, I shouted to one of the other students to call a teacher from the nearby faculty lounge. The reactions from the two faculty members who responded were similar to those of the students. Finally the director arrived and was able to contact the girl's parents and to arrange for her transportation to and evaluation at a nearby emergency facility.

Later that day, I repeatedly heard from the faculty about how wonderful it was that I had been with the student as she convulsed. I responded by saying, "What would have happened if I had been out of the building that day?" It is my premise that the first aid I rendered could have been done by anyone; it was not my exclusive territory because I was the school nurse. I used the information gained about the school community that day to plan and to deliver an inservice on epilepsy to the faculty and to arrange for all faculty to take a cardiopulmonary resuscitation class at school. I also spoke with the students about epilepsy and answered their questions.

It is hard to evaluate the effectiveness of my interventions because we did not have a similar incident at school that year. I am secure in saying, however, that the faculty were at least better equipped to deal with a medical emergency because of the health classes. How they would have responded had there actually been another emergency I do not know.

Situation C: Groups

Students at Jones School participated in several different groups. As previously mentioned, the focus of the nurse's group was the physical and psychological changes of pregnancy, labor, and delivery. Students also participated in a group session with the social worker weekly. This group focused on the student's relationships with her family and with the father of the baby and the student's current plans for her infant.

Frequently the social worker and I found it necessary to spend several hours weekly sharing information derived from our groups. Sometimes I would learn about a health problem that the student was experiencing. The social worker usually wasn't aware of the situation. In the same way, the social worker often learned new information not known to me.

I decided to see how the students felt about the group. A survey revealed that they thought they spent too much time in groups. The survey also showed that the students were disappointed when the nurse's group (10 weeks in length) finished before the delivery of their baby. Individual students seemed to visit me with increased frequency. Student responses varied about the social worker's group. Some felt that this group should be optional.

I approached the school social worker with a plan to combine our groups in order to be more comprehensive and efficient. I thought we would do well co-leading a group that dealt with the physical, social, and emotional issues of pregnancy. The combined group would also allow us to decrease some of our weekly coordinating time. The social worker heartily supported the plan. We discussed our proposal with the other faculty and staff. They, too, supported the plan. Our proposal was initiated the following school year—very successfully, I might add.

The combined social worker/nurse groups definitely were a more holistic approach to dealing with the total needs of students. The time that the social worker and the nurse needed to meet to coordinate was decreased considerably. The time spent in groups each week by students was reduced as well. The new group was received very positively by most students and has continued at Jones School.

Situation D: Labor and Delivery

During "Nurse's Group," students frequently talked about labor and delivery and the anticipation of the birth of their babies. My assessment from my first groups was that the students had much need for support from the faculty at Jones. In informal discussion with the faculty and staff at Jones, I learned that there was no clear way to learn when students delivered their babies. Often a day or two would pass before the school would hear of the birth.

It seemed to me that the adolescents needed a way to inform the staff at Jones about the birth of their babies. I decided to ask the students to call me when their babies were born. I gave them my home and office phone numbers and made it clear that evening and weekend phone calls were acceptable. One of the thoughts behind my request was that I wanted to reinforce each student's self-esteem. I wanted the students to know that I, and the other faculty and staff at Jones, cared about them. I also wanted to share in their excitement at this special moment in their lives.

I didn't expect the responses I received. Nearly everyone who delivered that school year called. In fact, one weekend while I was out of town, six students left messages about the births of their babies. Whenever possible, I visited the students and their babies at the maternity units of the local hospitals. I found these visits to be an appropriate time to review the events of labor and delivery with the adolescent and to focus on how she was doing now, postdelivery. I also reinforced the procedure the student should follow to request homebound tutoring before returning to school. I sometimes contacted the new mother's PHN to let her know about the birth of the baby.

It is hard to measure how the health of the community changed because of the interventions noted. I would like to think that the human contact received at this special moment of their lives was meaningful.

RECOMMENDATIONS

Community assessment is an essential strategy for nurses working with special populations. It is necessary for the nurse to assess and to diagnose accurately the population she is serving. In order to improve the health of the individual school community, the nurse must determine its needs and plan appropriate interventions. When community assessment techniques are employed, the health status of the community improves, and the satisfaction of the nurse improves as well.

CHAPTER 12

THE OCCUPATIONAL HEALTH NURSE IN AN INDUSTRIAL COMMUNITY

JO McNEIL, R.N., M.N.

The occupational health nurse has a unique role in providing health services to a community. Each industry or business comprised of employees, management, and the work site can be considered a community client. This chapter describes how an occupational health nurse developed a program based on an assessment using existing data regarding the health needs of the working population and responded to a request for assistance by a specific industrial community.

The Occupational Health Specialist at Seattle-King County Health Department (Seattle, Washington) is a person who has a baccalaureate degree in nursing, occupational health, industrial hygiene, or a closely related field and a master's degree in occupational health or a closely related field. In this agency, the Occupational Health Specialist is a nurse who develops and conducts occupational health programs by screening workers for job-related illness or injury, conducts educational programs to reduce adverse health and safety effects in the workplace, and promotes improved health practices such as preventive health behavior. This nurse specialist directs program staff, promotes occupational health contracts, coordinates work, evaluates outcomes, and directly provides many of the screenings and other services.

PROBLEM IDENTIFICATION

At the request of the mayor and the city council, members of the health department and others developed the *Seattle Health Policy*, which provides general guidelines for community health services. The 1981 *Seattle Health Policy* is based on the national health policy known as *Healthy People: The Surgeon General's Report on Health Promotion and Disease Prevention*, published in 1979. Both the national and local health policy statements are supported by extensive epidemiological and demographic data analysis. Review of the analysis of the data and the resulting recommendations revealed that the leading causes of death for the adult population are cancer, heart disease, and stroke. Smoking, stress, hypertension, high cholesterol levels, diabetes, overweight, and lack of exercise were identified as the major risk factors in the development of both heart disease and stroke.[1,2] The occupational health nurse in this health department uses the *Seattle Health Policy* as a guide in planning programs.

The focus of the Seattle-King County Occupational Health Program is the working population not served by a resident occupational health nurse. Large businesses usually employ occupational nurses. However, with most of the workers in this country working in small companies who have not yet seen the advantage of part-time or hourly occupational health nurses, 79 percent of workers in private, nonfarm businesses do not have access to such a nurse.[3] The major portion of this population ranges in age from 18 to 65 years.

Health problems in the work arena were identified and ranked in importance by the National Institute of Occupational Safety and Health (NIOSH) using the following criteria: 1) frequency of occurrence, 2) severity of disease to the individual, and 3) the disease's amenability to prevention:

1. Occupational lung disease
2. Musculoskeletal injuries
3. Occupational cancers (other than lung)
4. Amputations
5. Cardiovascular diseases
6. Disorders of reproduction caused by occupational exposures
7. Neurotoxic disorders caused by occupational exposures
8. Noise-induced hearing loss
9. Dermatologic conditions caused by occupational exposures
10. Psychologic disorders.[4]

Screening for chronic health problems in the work arena has been supported by the Seattle-King County Health Department as well as by NIOSH. Seattle-King County Health Department chose the following criteria to determine its priorities for screening for chronic health problems: 1) appropriate follow up is available, 2) early diagnosis is demonstrated to improve the cure rate and for quality of life, and 3) screening is coupled with appropriate information and education.

In a review of data related to efforts to prevent cardiovascular diseases, the following factors seemed significant. One in five persons between the ages of 25 and 64 have elevated blood pressure.[5] Large numbers of persons with hypertension die or are disabled by stroke and heart disease. Diet, exercise, coping with stress, and drug therapy are some of the many types of treatment to reduce blood

---

pressure and the potential for stroke. One such program increased the number of employees adhering to treatment from 40 percent adhering to treatment with 36 percent under control to 77 percent adhering to treatment with 82 percent under adequate control.[6] Therefore, although cardiovascular disease is ranked fifth in importance by NIOSH, it was chosen as a high priority based on the local health department criteria.

RESOURCE ANALYSIS

When it was determined that hypertension was a potential problem in the work force, an analysis of existing resources was undertaken to identify agencies currently providing high blood pressure control services in this area. The Seattle Occupational Health Committee (SOHC) was initiated in 1981 to complement and to support existing occupational health endeavors. A look at nonprofit agencies and the services they provide indicated that a collaborative high blood pressure control program was not going to compete with other agencies already active in this area. Four other agencies indicated they were interested or were doing hypertension screening. The American Heart Association and the Red Cross were already involved in screening programs in small companies using volunteers. A third provider was Providence Medical Center Impact-Health Promotion Program, which was primarily interested in more comprehensive wellness screening programs. Visiting Nurse Service was also considering development of some type of screening program. Figure 12-1 is a directory of occupational health services provided by agencies in the Seattle-King County area.[7]

A review of existing data and available services constituted the assessment which identified hypertension control as a high priority for the Occupational Health Program at the Seattle-King County Health Department. The more popular health assessment and wellness programs seemed to reach the healthiest of the workers, take much more of the worker's company time, and often cost about two and a half times more than the high blood pressure control programs. The latter tend to reach out for the high-risk clients and follow-up services are for those at greater risk of illness. Smoking and overeating are frequently associated with increased blood pressure. Blood pressure control programs provide an opportunity to approach these more sensitive issues.

PROGRAM DEVELOPMENT

Once it was determined that the health department would offer this program, as a district administrator responsible for the development of occupational health services, I notified industries in King County of the services available through

		Occupational Disease				Health Surveillance			Worksite Evaluation				Information					Education & Training					Research			Individual Counseling				Group Education Topics				Screening			Referral & Consultation		
Page No.	Agency	Diagnosis	Follow-up	Rehabilitation	Evaluation per Phone	Pre-employment	Specialized Screening: Lead, Asbestos, Noise	Customized Screening By Arrangement	Walk Through	Environmental Sampling	Laboratory Services	Health Hazard Evaluation	Regulations and Standards	Toxicological Health Effects	Referral and Community Services	Professional Legal Resp. & Limitations	Workplace Exposure Controls	For Managers	For Workers	For Health Prof.	For Unions	Manpower Resources	Occupational Disease Registry	Customized Epidemiological Studies		Lifestyle and Health	Substance Abuse	Stress Management	Pregnancy	Lifestyle and Health	Substance Abuse	Protective Work Practices	Stress Management	Diabetes	Hypertension	Cancer	Community Resources	Technical Assistance	Program Planning
5	AMERICAN CANCER SOCIETY																													✓	✓					✓			
7	AMERICAN HEART ASSOCIATION														✓															✓					✓		✓	✓	✓
9	AMERICAN LUNG ASSOCIATION												✓	✓	✓				✓	✓							✓										✓		
10	AMERICAN RED CROSS																	✓	✓	✓	✓								✓						✓				
12	CHILDREN'S ORTHOPEDIC HOSP. POISON CONTROL CENTER				✓								✓	✓	✓																								
13	DSHS OCCUPATIONAL HEALTH UNIT							✓						✓	✓	✓	✓			✓		✓		✓	✓												✓	✓	✓
15	HARBORVIEW MEDICAL CENTER OCCUPATIONAL MEDICINE CLINIC	✓	✓		✓		✓	✓	✓			✓	✓	✓	✓	✓			✓	✓	✓			✓	✓													✓	
18	INJURED WORKERS ORGANIZATION		✓	✓					✓				✓		✓	✓		✓	✓	✓	✓	✓				✓		✓		✓			✓				✓	✓	✓
19	PROVIDENCE MEDICAL CENTER IMPACT-HEALTH PROMOTION PROG.														✓				✓							✓	✓	✓		✓	✓		✓		✓		✓	✓	✓
20	PUGET SOUND HEALTH SYSTEMS AGENCY								✓																					✓							✓	✓	✓
21	SEATTLE KING COUNTY HEALTH DEPARTMENT					✓	✓	✓	✓				✓	✓	✓				✓	✓	✓					✓	✓	✓	✓	✓	✓	✓	✓		✓		✓	✓	✓
23	UNITED WAY OF KING COUNTY													✓				✓	✓	✓	✓									✓	✓		✓				✓		
24	UNIVERSITY OF WASHINGTON DEPT. OF ENVIRONMENTAL HEALTH								✓	✓	✓	✓	✓	✓	✓			✓	✓	✓				✓															
25	UNIVERSITY OF WASHINGTON EDUCATIONAL RESOURCE CENTER												✓	✓	✓		✓	✓	✓	✓	✓	✓		✓	✓					✓	✓	✓	✓				✓	✓	✓
26	VISITING NURSE SERVICES OF SEATTLE KING COUNTY		✓	✓									✓	✓	✓			✓	✓		✓					✓	✓	✓	✓	✓	✓	✓	✓	✓	✓		✓	✓	✓
27	WASHINGTON OCCUPATIONAL HEALTH RESOURCE CENTER												✓	✓	✓		✓		✓	✓	✓											✓					✓	✓	

FIGURE 12-1. Occupational services and agencies, Seattle, King County, WA. From Seattle Occupational Health Committee: *Check into Occupational Health*. A directory of services in the Seattle, King County area. Seattle, WA, December, 1982.

the health department. During the process I was excited to receive a request to supervise the screening and to do the follow-up services for a large high blood pressure control program in a local shipbuilding company. One of the most positive aspects of this request was that it was the president of the company who saw a need and instructed his safety and health director to implement it. Administrative support is a key factor to a successful program.

Seattle-King County Health Department joined the existing collaborative efforts of the American Heart Association and the King County High Blood Pressure Control Program in a team effort to provide a comprehensive program. The health department became involved with these agencies through informal networking among nurses interested in worksite hypertension programs. With a small program that could expand by using hourly public health nurses, the health department was an appropriate agency to provide quality service and confidentiality requested by the workers, union, and company management.

The local shipbuilding company can be conceptualized as a community. In this instance, worker interaction was evident as I watched several thousand workers and their families participate in launching of "their" ship in mid 1983. As she slid down the greased skids and splashed into Puget Sound, thousands of colorful balloons filled the sky and danced to the military band and cheers of the workers. They helped put this ship together and she was completed ahead of schedule. They were a proud team—a happy community that day.

Shipbuilding is a competitive business, and the job can be stressful. This company, as others, hires and fires as needed to meet the contracts. Last year they had about 2000 workers and this year over 3000. This company is part of the 1 percent of companies in the United States that employ over 500 people. Although this company did not meet the criteria established for participation in the program on the basis of size, it did not have an occupational health nurse and showed interest in being involved. Therefore it was included in the services provided by the agency.

The company has three worksites within a few miles of each other. Workers can be transferred between the sites frequently, which adds to the complexity for the nurse or others providing follow-up services. The company is made up of skilled workers, who may come and go. The hourly workers are an average age of 42.3 years, and the salaried workers are 43.5 years. The workers are unionized, and there is competition for the jobs in an 11 percent unemployment climate. Caucasions make up 85 percent of the workers. The minorities are only 6 percent black, 6 percent Asians, 2 percent Hispanic, and 1 percent other ethnic groups. Male workers are 88 percent and female workers are 12 percent of the work force.

Program Goals

The goals of the screening program were that by 1985, 70 percent of the employees participating in the follow-up portion of the program should realize improvement in their blood pressure or maintain a controlled status, and, of those, that

60 percent should achieve/maintain control. Blood pressure evaluations are divided into the following groupings of diastolic blood pressure (DBP):

Status of Elevation Determined by Diastolic Blood Pressure (DBP)
Group 1   DBP $\geq$ 115
Group 2   DBP $\geq$ 96 $\leq$ 114
Group 3   DBP $\geq$ 90 $\leq$ 95
Group 4   DBP $<$ 90

Criteria for improvement of blood pressure status is a change to at least the next lower group (for example, change from Group 2 to Group 3 as defined above) over the period of participation. Achievement or maintenance of a control status is defined as Group 4 (DBP $<$ 90).

Methodology

The High Blood Pressure Control Program is divided into the following five parts: publicity, education, screening/referral, follow up, and rescreening/referral. Publicity is done by the company with technical assistance from the planning committee (a representative from each of the collaborating agencies) to heighten awareness of the program through flyers, posters, articles in the company newsletter, articles in the daily newspaper, notices in paycheck envelopes, and discussions at the work group meetings.

The education is done in groups of 10 to 16 workers and their supervisor. These are scheduled by the company and last about 15 minutes. A short film and question-and-answer session covers the meaning, impact, methods, and benefits of controlling high blood pressure as well as specific risk factors such as smoking, overweight, and high sodium intake. Stressed at this session is the confidentiality of each worker's health status information. This is done on company time, as is the follow-up service. Immediately after the education session, blood pressure screening is offered in an adjoining space by a team of nurses. Having blood pressure actually taken is a voluntary action on the part of the worker.

The mass screening is held each fall, and the guidelines approved by the American Heart Association are used. Nurse screeners are trained each year by the American Heart Association. Workers are told what their blood pressure reading is. A brochure addressing risk factors, healthy life styles, and means of controlling blood pressure are available at this point and questions are answered. If rescreening is needed, the client makes an appointment and fills out an appointment reminder.

Follow up/tracking is done using the Washington State Department of Social and Health Services' computerized Hypertension Information System. The King County High Blood Pressure Control Program coordinates data input and analyzes the information which is often used as an evaluation tool. Those needing follow up are given an identification number. Monthly reports on status of each participant are sent to the health department. Follow-up visits to the Occupational Health Specialist continue as needed throughout the year.

Results

Progress toward the goal of reducing high blood pressure in this program may be demonstrated by comparing the results of the program in 1981-1982 with those in 1982-1983. The number of persons improving and/or maintaining control of their blood pressure increased significantly in the second program year. The number of individuals being followed at the time of evaluation and their status in relation to the criteria established is listed below.

	1981–1982	1982–1983
Total Screened	1,227	2,569
Follow-up Participants	389	829
Percent controlled at initial screening	5.4%	12.7%
Percent improved/controlled	40.9%	54.2%
Percent controlled	30.9%	40.8%

The increase in number screened the second year was a result of an overall increase in employees. The proportion of employees participating in the program remained essentially the same. The significant change from year one to year two was the increase in the percentage of participants improving and/or maintaining control. This increase indicated progress toward the program goals.

Additional useful information related to hypertension was obtained. Workers being followed for elevated blood pressure included a large number of smokers and an even greater number of overweight persons. This information was taken at the time of screening and manually tabulated for the risk group.

	Company Employees in Follow Up	U.S. Adult Population
Smoke cigarettes	42.5%	29%
Overweight	44.9%	25%

SUMMARY

As a result of the screening program, the following general recommendations were made:
1. Continue this high blood pressure control program in the same format.
2. Intensify information and education components of the program particularly in smoking and overweight.
3. Systematize the reporting regarding program progress.

The initial findings gain importance when considering that all the company workers had health insurance. All improvement seen through this program is an improvement over the community care available. Worksite occupational health services may be one of the only ways to provide services supportive enough to help the client control blood pressure. In the words of one employee with a history of stroke and heart disease whose blood pressure went from 176/116 to 126/86, this program acted as a "watchdog" in the most positive sense. Over several months, the continuing motivation of the nurses' monitoring and counselling helped this worker establish a medication regimen, reduce weight by 30 pounds, and get into an exercise program. The client's success spilled over to her two overweight daughters. A nursing role such as that used in this program can provide a comprehensive approach because a public health nurse is prepared to assist the client and physician with medication problems and to provide general counselling regarding diet and other necessary life style changes.

With a company of 3000 employees more aware of the tremendous costs of uncontrolled high blood pressure and the potential for successful control of the disease it is estimated that some 10,000 people in the community heard about some aspect of the program. The collaboration of the four agencies provided increased visibility in the community, and the networking increased the possibility of contracting with other companies for a high blood pressure control program. Depending on the staffing, the cost to the company can be as low as $5 per employee for this service for a year. Working with a company as a client, a preventive impact can be obtained for a small amount of money.

Once the company recognizes the skills of the occupational health nurse, it will take advantage of this type of professional and hire one. This was indeed the outcome of this project. The occupational health nurse I had originally hired in the health department was hired by the company full time to replace one of the safety and health team members who retired from the shipbuilding company. For other companies who have not had experience with occupational health nurses, it may take more creative marketing approaches to sell the idea. The high blood pressure control program may be the best tool because it offers many benefits to a company at a low cost. A few of the expected outcomes of such a program are increased productivity, increased morale, decreased costs for illness, decreased time lost for illness and medical office visits, decreased loss of staff from disability and premature death. In the next few years, many worksite communities will need to be assessed, and occupational health nursing services will be provided to the workers. When the percentage of workers with access to an occupational health nurse increases beyond the current 21 percent, the impact on the health of the 18-to-64 age group could be tremendous.

The preceding example views the work arena as a community client. It also demonstrates how organization and analysis of existing data can be used as the assessment process. In this instance, collection of additional information was not necessary. Existing data were sufficient to support program planning.

REFERENCES

1. SEATTLE DIVISION, SEATTLE-KING COUNTY DEPARTMENT OF PUBLIC HEALTH: *Seattle Health Policy*. April 1981, pp 27–31.

2. US DEPARTMENT OF HEALTH, EDUCATION AND WELFARE: *Healthy People*. The Surgeon General's Report on Health Promotion and Disease Prevention. PHS Publication #79-550717, Washington, DC, 1979, pp 56–59.

3. US LABOR DEPARTMENT: *Occupational Injuries and Illness by Industry, 1972*. Bulletin #1830, Washington, DC, 1974.

4. NATIONAL INSTITUTE OF OCCUPATIONAL SAFETY AND HEALTH: *Occupational Safety and Health Report*. September 1, 1983, Vol 13, No 14, p 324.

5. US DEPARTMENT OF HEALTH AND HUMAN SERVICES: *Health: United States 1980 with Prevention Profile*. PHS Publication #81-1232, Washington, DC, 1981, p 35.

6. LAPOINTE, MH AND ORMSBY, P: *Case study in high BP control: Mass mutual life insurance company*. Occupational Health Nursing, November 1981, pp 39–40.

7. SEATTLE OCCUPATIONAL HEALTH COMMITTEE: *Check Into Occupational Health*. A directory of services in the Seattle–King County area. Seattle, WA, 1982, pp 16–17.

CHAPTER 13

THE COMMUNITY AS A CLIENT: A CASE STUDY IN INFECTION CONTROL PRACTICE

KATHERINE HILL CHAVIGNY, R.N., Ph.D., F.A.C.E.

An assessment of a community can be as varied and singular as an individual client assessment. The first step in the nursing process (assessment) evokes models for different approaches according to client need. Nursing models are methods to approach and assist assessment and implementation of other steps in the nursing process. Process requires content, just as "how" to assess requires "what" to assess.[1] For an individual, holistic care connotes substance or content of the process—the physical, social, psychological, and spiritual areas to assure inclusive nursing care services. Using process and content, patient/client needs can be highly individualized.

The assessment of a community is similar: Various approaches can be used to implement a method for assessment. However, when the community is the client, the characteristics of the target population and the type of problem dictate the most desirable and practical methodologic technique. For instance, Programmed Evaluation Review Technique (PERT) may be useful when terminal objectives can be clearly identified, in advance, to help guide the assessment. Systems analysis is also a useful approach, especially when the community of need, the subset of a population requiring care, must be linked with the reciprocal subgroup of providers or significant others who are the community of solution.[2] These approaches are method oriented. In other words, they describe how to do the assessment but do not address what needs to be included in the assessment of a community. The distinction is important: in individualized nursing care, the model for assessment may change, but the subject areas for the holistic approach remain the same. Similarly, in community assessment, the approach or method may change. Woolsey and Lawrence recommend fundamental content or subject areas which remain constant.[3] Thus a community assessment includes the collection of five basic sets of information for every population. Other authors have identified content areas necessary for an accurate assessment; but Woolsey and Lawrence have an advantage of being succinct, inclusive, and simple. Their approach also evokes an effective method, the epidemiologic method, as a process-oriented means of collecting information. Another advantage is that through identifying what needs to be the content of an assessment of a community, the nurse is directed to information which might be readily and easily available from libraries and local departments of public health. This assures that the assessment process will be directed to gathering and organizing information not available from alternative sources.

Woolsey and Lawrence recommend five basic types of information for a complete community assessment.[4] The five types of data are

1. Counts of people
2. Measures of health status
3. Health services received by the population
4. Health services and resources in the population including manpower, facilities, and political-economic support
5. State of the environment.

Counts of people may be information gathered by the decennial census or may be available from nursing agency records. This information is the number of people, ill and well, in the target population. Measures of health status are the rates and ratios published by the National Center for Health Statistics and local departments. The assessment of a smaller community often involves gathering estimates of the number of people who are ill with one or more diagnoses. This is called numerator data, and they are used to compute the rate, the basic epidemiologic statistic.

The records for health services received are found at many locations in the community. Clinics, hospitals, and nursing agencies have ongoing lists of patients receiving care and, within the limits of preserving patient confidentiality, will share information. Community resources regarding health manpower and available facilities are sometimes less available than other kinds of data. Often the chamber of commerce and university departments of nursing, medicine, and allied professions have statistics on personnel available to deliver health care needs in the community. Finally, the state of the environment can be assessed not only to identify exposures to health risks—such as air pollution, water, and sewage facilities—but also transportation required for access to services. Ecologic and geographic relationships of high-risk subpopulations are also part of the environmental information.

In an ideal situation, the assessment of a community may involve the collection and assembly of these data. Due care must be given to validity of sources and the time frame to which the information refers. Most frequently, however, the target population is specific—much too specific for any previous records to be available for reference; for example, a group of school-age children of migrant workers. Often the assessment is made to determine if resources are available for services or to quantify a discrete need, such as the number of clients with undetected hypertension in a population of Vietnam refugees. It is unlikely that records have already been compiled for these smaller groups or communities. Nonetheless, it is an advantage to look for statistics regarding the five types of information to determine if they are already available or if the assessment needs to gather new data. It should be clear that counts are essential to successful community assessment. The community to be assessed comprises denominator data. The problems within the community are numerator data, so that measures of health, such as the rate, can be generated. The epidemiologic method as a problem-solving approach has been discussed in Chapter 3. It is a very useful approach in community assessment and is the process used in the following case study. The discussion will emphasize the use of Woolsey and Lawrence as content areas for assessment of a community.

CASE STUDY

The following case study will illustrate the way the five basic requirements guide and direct the activities of assessment. The community setting was a university hospital. A hospital is an agency of the extramural community and contributes to control of disease in the population as a whole. The purpose of the assessment was first, to estimate the immunization status of all staff and personnel in the hospital complex; second, to estimate the cost of a project to immunize the employees; and third, to identify a method of providing immunization for the target population. Although the need for the assessment had been recognized by the hospital administration for some time, the problem was precipitated by an outbreak of diphtheria on the nearby Indian reservation during an interstate powwow. Over 300 members of the tribes had gathered from four states. The outbreak began with eight diagnosed cases of diphtheria. As the meeting dispersed, the infection was carried back to home reservations and urban centers close to the reservations. New cases occurred, and patients with diphtheria from the skid-row area were admitted to the university hospital caring for medically underserved groups. Unfortunately, it rapidly became apparent that a cadre of RNs and other staff with up-to-date immunity to diphtheria were unavailable to maintain around-the-clock care of these very ill patients.

The protection of staff from occupational hazards was the responsibility of the infection control committee, a multidisciplinary representation of all the hospital disciplines, including nursing. The committee chair was head of public health and preventive medicine. The infection control nurse executed the policies of the committee. An emergency meeting of the infection control committee was called, in which it was decided to survey the hospital to assess the need for an immunization program.

The community assessment was undertaken by the infection control practitioner (ICP). The role of the ICP is the surveillance of the hospital community for the early detection and prevention of nosocomial infection and occupational health hazards. The ICP applies the policies of the multidisciplinary infection control committee and was, in fact, the public health nurse of this intramural community. Part of the function of the ICP is the continuous assessment of the hospital, and it was, therefore, part of the role to conduct the community assessment for status of immunity for communicable diseases of personnel and patients.

First, the target population had to be clearly identified. It was not clear whether patients were to be included in the group or whether the population was to be restricted to nurses, physicians, and direct care personnel. Administration determined that physicians and medical students would update their immunizations through the student health service and/or private care. Inpatient immunizations were a more difficult responsibility because they had to be administered according to physician prescription for each patient, owing to complexity of the diagnoses and therapeutic regimens. It was decided that this problem would be resolved on a physician-client basis for all admissions. The remaining subgroup consisted of all nursing staff and support personnel, including engineering, housekeeping, laboratory and dietary services. This group represented the target population. Counts of employees were obtained from the director of nursing services as well as the heads of the other departments. The total number of people in the subpopulation was almost 1500 persons, and this constituted the "community of concern," or target group.

The assessment began with the quantification of the levels of immunity in these employees. A questionnaire was sent to all units and floors of the hospital as well as to all support departments. A meeting of head nurses was called, and their cooperation was requested in filling and returning the questionnaires for nursing staff on the floors, clinics, and intensive care units of the hospital. The completed questionnaires were then collected during daily ward and departmental rounds by the ICP. The most difficult nursing staff to contact were those on the 11:00 PM to 7:00 AM shift, and a visit by the ICP to the floors during shift change facilitated the collection of the completed questionnaires. Also, additional forms were left at each station to compensate for loss and misplacement of the forms. Owing in large part to the diligent efforts of the head nurses and departmental heads, a 95 percent return on this questionnaire survey was accomplished.

The questionnaire requested time and dates of vaccination or surveillance for poliomyelitis, rubella, tuberculosis (TB), and hepatitis A and B as well as diphtheria and tetanus. Members of the staff who were unsure of their health status gave permission for the ICP to contact their private physicians to verify information. In the survey, the total number of respondents was 1425. A computer card was made out for each respondent, and the information was tallied. Only 35 percent of all respondents had had complete immunizations for diphtheria and tetanus, 10 percent had had rubella and 8 percent poliomyelitis vaccinations. State law no longer required yearly TB surveillance of hospital personnel, but only 20 percent of current employees reported that they had received a tuberculin skin test (PPD) or x-ray examination within the last 12 months. It was obvious to the committee that in order to update the immunization status of this community, an immediate full-scale immunization program was required. The assessment continued.

Information was needed concerning the environment and the resources available to deliver the program. It became apparent that the health service did not have enough staff in addition to their ongoing duties to accomplish the task. The nursing supervisors were understandably reluctant to divest the floors of the hospital of RNs in order that they could go to a central location for immunizations. The geographic location of the different departments was spread throughout many buildings across the university campus. An outreach program seemed the best method of solution. The ICP and the secretary of the Infection Control Program would rotate through all the hospital floors and other departments of the hospital. A meeting of head nurses was called to determine a feasible schedule; it was thought that a twice-daily visit to each floor at the turn of the shifts for 2 weeks would cause the least disruption of patient care. Departmental heads of other services decided that 2 consecutive days in each place would be the most feasible and effective organizational pattern.

Costs of the program were a relevant concern and were estimated from the questionnaires. The accounting department supplied current cost of diphtheria-tetanus vaccine, PPD, and x-ray examinations as cents per client. The university hospital administrators were informed of total costs, and a discussion of legal implications for failure to provide immunization to staff was detailed. The administration decided to fund the program except for rubella and poliomyelitis immunizations. After 2 weeks of an intensive outreach operation, all staff were offered immunizations at their place of work within the hospital community.

The assessment was not considered complete until a final quantification of the immune status of the community had been made. All vaccinations, PPD, and x-ray examination orders had been recorded and entered on the same computer card assigned to each employee after the receipt of the questionnaire. From these records, the number and types of procedures could be identified. These were numerator data. Administration provided the number of regular position employees half-time and over, a total of 1500 positions. This comprised the denominator data. Losses occurred from four sources:

1. Refusal to be included (10 percent of all contacts)
2. Terminated employees (these immunizations were not included in the analysis)
3. Employees not surveyed because of vacation, illness, or days off during the outreach to their department (estimated 10 percent)
4. Recently hired employees not included in initial questionnaire (estimated 5 percent of total positions).

The overall immune status in this population for diphtheria-tetanus was 71 percent. Seventy-five percent of all employees were surveyed for TB. From this time on, notice of recently hired employees were sent to the infection control practitioner, who held a once-a-week clinic to assure ongoing vaccination and surveillance of new employees. Soon after the completion of this program, three more cases of diphtheria were admitted to the hospital without hazard to employees or deprivation of nursing care to the patients.

SUMMARY

The hospital is a community. The case study describes a community assessment for a subgroup of employees at high risk for communicable diseases. It was necessary to include all members of the target population, and therefore it was not necessary to use any sampling procedure. The process used was epidemiologic and began with identifying a problem, collecting observations, analyzing data, and drawing conclusions. The content areas were defined by Woolsey and Lawrence. First, the need for an employee immunization was assessed, and then the effects of an immunization program were quantified. The situation was stabilized by providing ongoing surveillance for immunization status for new employees for nursing staff and support services.

REFERENCES

1. FITZPATRICK, J AND WHALL, A: *Conceptual Models of Nursing: Analysis and Application.* Robert J. Brady, Bowie, MD, 1983.

2. ARCHER, SE AND FLESHMAN, RP: *Community Health Nursing: Patterns and Practice,* ed 2. Duxbury Press, North Scituate, MA, 1979.

3. WOOLSEY, T AND LAWRENCE, P: *Moving ahead in health statistics.* Am J Public Health 59(10):1820, 1969.

4. Ibid, p 1821.

CHAPTER 14

A LEARNING EXPERIENCE FOR BACCALAUREATE NURSING STUDENTS

LINDA FELVER, R.N., M.A.
DONNA B. HAW, R.N., B.S.N.

Stethoscopes in use, four nursing students sat near a long table in the hall outside a high school classroom. Small clusters of high school students stood around the table, some of them using each others' backs as flat surfaces on which to fill out questionnaires. All available chairs and table space were occupied. Other students filtered through the hall, pausing to read a 10-foot-long poster on the wall behind the tables. "What is high blood pressure?" said the poster. "Seniors, have your blood pressure checked," said another sign. Many of them joined their fellow students in filling out the questionnaires and having their blood pressures taken by the student nurses. A similar scene was taking place in another hallway on the other side of the same high school.

Why did eight nursing students record over 200 blood pressure measurements that morning and then repeat the performance at another high school the next week? What was the motivating force behind the massive hypertension teaching poster? The baccalaureate nursing students were enrolled in Community Health Nursing at the Intercollegiate Center for Nursing Education in Spokane, Washington. One of their course requirements was completion of a community assessment group project. A research format for community assessment was an approach students could choose to fulfill this requirement. The scene described above was a portion of the community health research project planned and implemented by this small group of nursing students. This chapter will describe the research project from its inception to its completion (approximately 10 weeks) and demonstrate how the students' research project both fulfilled the course objectives and made a small impact on the health of the community.

DEVELOPMENT OF THE RESEARCH PROJECT

Eight community health nursing students sat somewhat bewildered about the choice in front of them. The students had been assigned to work together on a community assessment project. The choice was either a regular community assessment or a research format for the community assessment. The group decided to use the research format (Table 14-1).

For the first two weeks, progress was slow. Members verbalized a variety of ideas for the research project. Most ideas were thrown out based on the amount of group interest and the degree of complexity. A few members demonstrated knowledge of research methodology and statistics. Other group members began to look to them for leadership. Finally, on the third group meeting there was a general consensus that hypertension among adolescents would be an interesting topic to define further and to research. The group departed that day with the task of reviewing the literature on hypertension and related factors.

At the same time the group was developing a research project, it was also given the task of monitoring and evaluating the dynamics of its own group pro-

TABLE 14-1. Community Health Nursing Research Assignment

   I. Select a problem within a community
      A. Identify the purpose of study
      B. Identify the limits of study
      C. State significance of problem
         1. In general
         2. In nursing
      D. State need for investigation
  II. Review literature relating to problem
      A. Relate review to problem studied
      B. Clarify the problem
      C. Study previous research studies in light of stated hypothesis(es)
 III. State hypothesis(es)
      A. Describe in measurable terms
      B. State dependent and independent research hypothesis(es)
 IV. Identify procedure for validation of research hypothesis(es)
      A. Determine method of data collection
      B. State rationale for its appropriateness
      C. Describe validity and reliability of method used
  V. Analyze results of data
      A. Present findings objectively and accurately
      B. Draw conclusions from findings presented
 VI. Summarize
      A. Discuss objectivity and accuracy of research done
      B. State relevancy to community health nursing

Course material, N440, Community Health Nursing, Intercollegiate Center for Nursing Education.

cess. At every group meeting there was to be a recorder, and each member was to assume responsibility for commenting about the evolution of the group. During the first few meetings there was vying for the leadership role. Members tested the group limits by suggesting wild ideas. The group responded by taking on a serious committed attitude. It was soon established that the group would work hard and do a good job while completing the assignment.

With the specific area of study defined, the group quickly moved into the working phase. The first task was to identify specific hypotheses about hypertension and the population the group had decided to investigate. Members suggested factors that might affect a person's blood pressure. These suggestions stemmed from the review of literature as well as the members' own ideas. Hypertension was identified as the dependent variable, and 15 other factors such as obesity, salt intake, and a family history of hypertension were labeled independent variables. These factors were described in measurable terms in the form of hypotheses (Table 14-2).

Having defined the hypotheses, the group decided that a high school would be a readily defined community that would meet the requirements for an adolescent age group. To keep the study within a manageable size the community was further defined to include only the senior classes of two local high schools.

It became evident that the group needed to define hypertension and obesity in measurable terms. A local Spokane cardiologist and multiple references were consulted. The final decision was that a blood pressure reading of 135/90 or higher would be considered hypertensive. Obesity was defined as a weight greater than 20 percent of the designated weight based on a person's height and age.

Simultaneously the group was evolving into a very efficient, cohesive, working unit. Leadership was established and members readily exchanged ideas, information, and suggestions. Problem solving and decision making were active processes involving all group members. The group was determined to do the job well. There was a common goal among all members.

With hypertension and its possible related factors as the focus and members of the senior high-school class as the target community, the group devised a method of study. The group agreed that a questionnaire composed of all the factors listed in the hypotheses should serve as the assessment tool. This tool, in conjunction with the students' blood pressures, would provide the data necessary to test the hypotheses. The group decided the questionnaire should be composed of response category questions instead of open-ended questions, in order to structure the responses for ease in computing. A subgroup of nursing students devised the questionnaire and brought it back to the group for approval.

The questionnaire was piloted on some of the group members' adolescent siblings to test its utility and to expose any areas that might need revising. Indeed, there were useful suggestions from the pilot study. The revised questionnaire (Table 14-3) was taken to a local printer, and the cost for the printing was shared equally among the group members.

The next task at hand was to secure permission from the school officials.

TABLE 14-2. The Research Hypotheses

NULL HYPOTHESIS

There is no prevalence of hypertension among the high school seniors at two high schools in Spokane, WA.

ALTERNATIVE HYPOTHESES

There is a prevalence of hypertension among high school seniors.

The prevalence of hypertension is sex related.

The prevalence of hypertension is directly related to the presence of obesity.

The prevalence of hypertension is increased among the black portion of the population studied.

The prevalence of hypertension is decreased among persons who had not eaten before the blood pressure was taken.

The prevalence of hypertension is increased among persons who drink six or more cups of coffee per day.

The prevalence of hypertension is increased among persons who add salt to their food at the table.

The prevalence of hypertension is increased among smokers as compared with nonsmokers.

The prevalence of hypertension is increased among persons who consume alcoholic beverages as compared with nondrinkers.

The prevalence of hypertension is increased among persons who have family members with hypertension.

The prevalence of hypertension is increased among persons taking oral contraceptives.

The prevalence of hypertension is increased among persons taking amphetamines.

The prevalence of hypertension increases proportionally with the increase of subjectively perceived stress levels on the day of the study.

The prevalence of hypertension is increased in persons who subjectively perceive themselves to be highly pressured most or all of the time.

The prevalence of hypertension is decreased among persons who engage in school sports.

The prevalence of hypertension is decreased among persons who rate themselves as four or above on the questionnaire activity scale as compared with persons who rate themselves below four.

With a sample questionnaire and the proposed plan to take all the seniors' blood pressures, two group members went to the director of school health services. They were received very warmly by the director, also a nurse. She directed the members to the individual high school principals. At each respective high school, the principals expressed strong support and interest in the project. They readily made suggestions about the best way to have access to all the school seniors. At one high school, it was arranged for the group to be outside the auditorium following a senior class assembly. At the other school, the group was

TABLE 14-3. The Research Questionnaire

AGE: _____

SEX: male _____   female _____

HEIGHT: _____

WEIGHT: _____

ETHNIC ORIGIN (optional):

Caucasian _____   Native American _____
Black _____   Mexican American _____
Oriental _____   Other _____

EMPLOYED? Yes _____   No _____

DO YOU LIVE WITH (check all blocks that apply):

Father _____ Mother _____ Step-father _____ Step-mother _____ Guardian _____ Other _____

Number of sisters at home? _____   Number of brothers at home? _____

DID YOU EAT BREAKFAST THIS MORNING?   Yes _____   No _____

DID YOU DRINK COFFEE THIS MORNING?   Yes _____   No _____

HOW MANY CUPS OF COFFEE DO YOU DRINK EACH DAY?   Yes _____   No _____

DO YOU ADD SALT TO YOUR FOOD AT THE TABLE?   Yes _____   No _____

DO YOU SMOKE?   Yes _____   No _____

IF SO: Tobacco _____   Other _____

IF SO, HOW MUCH?: _____   HOW OFTEN?: _____

DO YOU DRINK ALCOHOL? _____   IF SO, HOW MUCH? _____   HOW OFTEN? _____

DO YOU HAVE A FAMILY DOCTOR? _____

IF YOU KNOW, WHAT IS YOUR BLOOD PRESSURE? _____

DO ANY OF YOUR FAMILY MEMBERS HAVE HIGH BLOOD PRESSURE? _____

WHAT MEDICATIONS ARE YOU CURRENTLY TAKING? _____

HAVE YOU EVER TAKEN HIGH BLOOD PRESSURE MEDICATION? _____

WHAT LEVEL OF STRESS DO YOU FEEL YOU ARE UNDER NOW?

High _____   Medium _____   Low _____

DO YOU FEEL HIGHLY PRESSURED?   Seldom _____   Most of the time _____
                                   Some of the time _____   All of the time _____

WHAT IS THE SOURCE OF THE MAJORITY OF YOUR PRESSURE?

Family _____   Friends _____
Sports _____   School _____
Work _____   Other _____

IN GENERAL, MY HEALTH IS: Excellent _____   Good _____   Fair _____   Poor _____

DO YOU PARTICIPATE IN SCHOOL SPORTS?   Yes _____   No _____

IF SO, WHICH SPORTS, HOW MUCH, AND HOW OFTEN? _____

WHAT OTHER FORMS OF EXERCISE DO YOU DO? _____

TABLE 14-3. The Research Questionnaire—*continued*

WHERE ARE YOU ON THE ACTIVITY SCALE?

0	3	6
Inactive	Moderately Active	Extremely Active

ARE YOU EXPERIENCING ANY OF THE FOLLOWING SYMPTOMS AT THIS TIME?

Dizziness _____
Headache _____
Awareness of heart beat _____
Blurred vision _____

IF SO, IS THIS A FREQUENT OCCURRENCE FOR YOU? _____

COMMENTS:

THANK YOU FOR YOUR TIME.

invited to the senior health classes. Both schools requested a copy of the analyzed data, and at one of the high schools, the health teacher took a particular interest in the project. He requested the nursing students to do some teaching about hypertension in addition to their data collection. This request for teaching would serve as a method for the group to meet many of the project's objectives as well as many of the community health course objectives.

It was now time to plan the logistics of the data collection. The group subdivided into smaller groups of two or three members and addressed such tasks as securing the equipment that would be needed, devising the specific teaching format, constructing the visual aids, and finalizing the specific dates and times of the group's meetings with the senior high school students. Within a week all the tasks were accomplished and the group was ready to go out and meet their chosen community.

IMPLEMENTATION OF THE RESEARCH PROJECT

Data Collection

Dressed in street clothes and wearing their school of nursing name tags, the group members were separated into two teams located just outside the entrances to the auditorium. Posters hanging overhead invited students to have their blood pressures checked. The teams were eagerly awaiting the arrival of the senior students. This was the setting at the first high school. In the auditorium, the senior class of students was gathered for an assembly. It was at the end of this class meeting that the seniors were given an explanation of the nursing project and were invited to participate in the blood pressure screening.

Soon each area was bustling with students at various stages of the screening process. First, the students approached the table stacked with questionnaires, pens and pencils, and boxes to deposit the finished questionnaires. Each was instructed to take a questionnaire, to answer all the questions, and to return to have a nursing student take his or her blood pressure. Numerous desks and chairs were available for the participants to complete the questionnaires and to have their blood pressures taken. When the students returned with the completed questionnaires, they were asked to keep their responses confidential. Then a nursing student paired up with a senior student, had the student sit in one of the chairs, took the blood pressure, and recorded it on the back side of the respective questionnaire. Each senior was informed of the blood pressure reading, and if the reading was greater than 135/90, the students were asked to have the blood pressure retaken in 5 minutes. The students were asked to have the blood pressure retaken in 5 minutes. The students were then instructed to deposit their questionnaires into one of the collection boxes on the table.

The response was better than the group had anticipated. Not only were the students interested, but a number of teachers asked to have their blood pressures checked. The group was willing to take anyone's blood pressure but was careful not to include them in the study. Many questions about the significance of an elevated blood pressure and how to prevent hypertension were brought up by the students on an individual basis. Throughout the project, group members explained what a blood pressure reading described, the risks of a prolonged high blood pressure, and possible factors that were thought to influence a person's blood pressure. These informal teaching sessions usually ended in the promotion of basic preventative, healthful patterns of living, including daily exercise, good nutrition, and routine check-ups with a professional health care provider. Nursing students advised seniors with two repeated elevated blood pressures to contact their physicians and to report the elevated blood pressures.

At the second high school, the arrangements for the group to screen the seniors were somewhat different. The group was invited to attend the health classes that were mandatory for all senior students. They were not only given the opportunity to complete their project but were also asked to teach the students about high blood pressure and its prevention. The format of having the students complete the questionnaires and having their blood pressures recorded was the same as at the previous high school. The difference was in the formalized teaching presentation that occurred after the screening. The group used a simplistic poster to help illustrate the meaning of the two numbers that composed a blood pressure reading. Then, once the students understood this basic concept, individual group members described the significance of an elevated blood pressure, factors that were thought to put individuals at risk for hypertension, and ways to reduce the possibility of developing hypertension. During the presentation the students were encouraged to ask questions and to verbalize their concerns. The time spent in the classes passed quickly for the group. The senior students were actively involved in the learning process. They asked many questions, not only in relation to their own health but also in regard to other family members. At the same time, group members were striving to present the information in an interesting yet factual way. The intent was to emphasize that hypertension was a problem that existed in the student's own age group and that by being aware and educated about the disease, it could be prevented or at least controlled at an early stage. Group members alternated in the teaching role and often would call upon one another for assistance to best address the specific issue of discussion. The group left the school feeling rewarded. They were given very positive feedback by the students and the two instructors. All in all, they had spent more than 12 hours directly involved with their designated population and now had access to the data they had set out to obtain. Additionally, they had been very active in educating the students.

Analysis of Data

Although most of the students in the group had no statistics background, one of the students was taking an introductory statistics course. After consultation with her statistics professor, she directed the data analysis.

One afternoon, the students gathered in a room with their 489 completed questionnaires, five hand calculators, and many large sheets of paper. One team of students compared heights and weights with the predetermined standards for obesity. Other teams of students tallied all the data from the questionnaires and checked each other's work. Using hand calculators, the Pearson product moment correlation coefficient was calculated for each possible relationship addressed in the null hypotheses.[1] The coefficients thus obtained were converted to standard normal deviates and compared with the previously established critical value of $|z| = 1.96$. (The critical value 1.96 had been chosen through consultation with a statistics professor. It indicates a p value of < 0.05, a statistically significant result.) All calculations were performed twice to check for accuracy. It was a long and arduous, but productive, afternoon.

PRESENTATION OF THE RESEARCH PROJECT

Planning of Class Presentation

Data and results now in hand, the students' attention turned toward planning the presentation of their project to their classmates and professors. How were they going to explain the entire project clearly in one hour while maintaining the attention and interest of the audience?

To ensure that all the relevant points were fully addressed, the students decided to use the Nursing 440, Community Health Nursing Rating Scale for Evaluation as the outline for the presentation (Table 14-4).

TABLE 14-4. Evaluation Criteria for the Community Health Nursing Research Assignment

	0	1	2	3	4	5
I. Problem selection A. Purpose and limits of study identified						
B. Significance of problem and rationale for investigation						
II. Review of literature A. Clearly relate to problem and hypothesis(es)						
III. Hypothesis A. State in measurable terms						
B. Dependent and independent variables identified						
IV. Validation A. Method used and rationale						
B. Validity and reliability						
V. Analysis A. Objective presentation of findings						
B. Valid conclusions						
VI. Summary A. Overall accuracy and value of research						
VII. Presenting team functions smoothly and cohesively						

Comments:

Rating Scale

Comprehensive coverage	Score 5
Lacks an essential point	Score 4
Moderate coverage of essential points	Score 3
Lacks several essential points	Score 2
Minimally covered	Score 1
Did not cover	Score 0

Course material, N440, Community Health Nursing, Intercollegiate Center for Nursing Education.

By this time, the group was very efficient at accomplishing necessary tasks and the process flowed smoothly. Individual students quickly volunteered to be responsible for the different sections of the presentation.

The question still remaining was how to maintain audience attention. Jubilant at having completed their research project, a few of the students suggested a dramatic opening to the presentation. They would portray a high school senior with multiple risk factors having her blood pressure taken on stage. The enthusiasm was contagious. Soon the presentation was loaded with visual aids and dramatic effects. This dramatic style was not only the answer to maintaining audience attention but also became a mechanism for group termination. The group goal had been fulfilled. The classroom presentation would be a form of shared celebration.

The Actual Presentation

As the class presentation was about to begin, one of the group members was busily stuffing her clothing with pillows to make herself appear obese. Other members were rushing about with armloads of picket signs, while still others were setting up props on the stage. Then the presentation began. Three students marched across the stage carrying the 10-foot hypertension teaching poster. Next, a cigarette-smoking, coffee-drinking, obese "high school senior" appeared on stage, followed by two student nurses who took her blood pressure.

Simultaneously, a group member was explaining the purpose and limits of the research project to the audience. She identified the twofold purpose of the study: first, to determine the prevalence of hypertension among the high school seniors at two local high schools and, second, to examine the relationship between hypertension and 15 independent variables. The audience was cautioned that generalizations from a research project must be confined to the population from which the sample was drawn, thus identifying the major limit of the study.

The focus of the presentation then shifted to the significance of the problem and the need for investigation. One of the students explained that although much research on hypertension had focused on the adult population, less attention had been given to hypertension in the adolescent population. Because nursing is involved with the promotion of health and the prevention of chronic illness, there was a need for further investigation of hypertension among the adolescent population.

The review of the literature[2-25] was presented by three teams of students. They discussed in turn the general causes and occurrence of hypertension, long-term effects of hypertension, specific factors suspected to influence blood pressure, and previous research on the prevalence of hypertension in adolescence.

''From the 24 references we used, which have just been discussed, we formulated the following hypotheses,'' said one of the group members. This sentence served as the introduction to a choral reading of the hypotheses. Solo voices, duets, and trios recited the 17 hypotheses in an orchestrated fashion. At the same time, a large scroll listing the hypotheses was being unrolled to serve as a visual cue.

The pace of the presentation accelerated as the dependent and independent variables were presented. The group members paraded around the stage carrying picket signs depicting the names of the variables. As the name of each variable was announced, the corresponding picket sign was firmly planted in a holder at the front of the stage. The friendly laughter in the room showed that audience response was enthusiastic.

The next topics addressed in the presentation were the method of data collection and the rationale for its appropriateness. The questionnaires were distributed to the audience while one of the group members explained that this assessment tool was a time- and energy-efficient way of obtaining the maximum amount of information needed to test the hypotheses. Additionally, the on-site measurement of blood pressures was the most direct way to obtain an accurate and current blood pressure.

After thus having described the rationale for appropriateness of the data collection method, the validity and reliability of the method were addressed. It was hoped that validity (accuracy) of the information reported on the questionnaires was increased by providing anonymity and by assuring the students that no school officials would have access to the questionnaires. The blood pressure measurements were considered valid because the nursing students recording them were proficient in the procedure and used the same protocol. In addition, the sphygmomanometers were calibrated directly before each data collection session. That the high blood pressures were truly elevated was supported by the fact that repetition of those blood pressures still showed values well above the pre-established criterion for hypertension. In addressing the issue of reliability, it was noted that in a preliminary blood pressure practice session among group members, inter-rater reliability was high.

The mood of the presentation became more serious as one of the group members presented the technical details of the data analysis and summarized the research findings. The formulas on the blackboard and the table of statistical findings required increased concentration from the audience.

TABLE 14-5. Prevalence of Hypertension in Two Spokane, Washington High Schools

SCHOOL	NUMBER SAMPLED	HYPERTENSIVE	NORMAL	PERCENT HYPERTENSIVE
A	215	7	208	3.26
B	274	7	267	2.55
Total	489	14	475	2.86

From the sample of 489 high school seniors at the two schools, 14 students (2.86 percent) were hypertensive, as defined by the preset criterion of blood pressure 135/90 or above (Table 14-5).

Statistical analysis of the questionnaire results produced the standard normal deviates reported in Table 14-6. Because of a printing error in the questionnaire, coffee intake data were sparse; coffee intake was therefore omitted from the computations. Owing to the small number of racial minorities sampled and the low incidence of reported usage of oral contraceptives and amphetamines, reliable estimates of correlations between each of these factors and the presence of hypertension could not be determined. Correlations were calculated between the presence of hypertension and each of the following factors separately: obesity, sex of student, no breakfast on the day of the study, salt intake, smoking of tobacco, smoking of tobacco plus "other," use of alcohol, family members with hypertension, stress level on the day of the study, perception of being highly pressured most or all the time, participation in school sports, and degree of physical activity.

TABLE 14-6. Summary of Statistical Analysis of Questionnaire Results

VARIABLE	$|z|$
Obesity	1.49
Sex of student	0.62
No breakfast	1.92
Salt intake	0.08
Use of tobacco	0.21
Use of tobacco and "other"	0.99
Use of alcohol	1.13
Family members with hypertension	2.92*
Stress level on day of study	
Medium vs low	0.84
High vs medium	0.35
Perception of being highly pressured most or all of the time	2.25*
School sports	0.28
Activity scale	0.17

*Indicates significant correlation ($|z| > 1.96$)

Of the factors studied, two were found to have significant correlation with the presence of hypertension: having family members with hypertension and the subjective perception of being highly pressured most or all the time. The presentor concluded that if the sample was truly representative of the high school seniors at the two Spokane high schools where the study was performed, then

1. The prevalence of hypertension among the high school seniors was 2.86 percent.
2. The occurrence of hypertension was increased among the high school seniors who had family members with hypertension and among those who subjectively perceived themselves to be highly pressured most or all of the time. The students noted that the 2.86 percent prevalance of hypertension obtained in this study was in accordance with the 3 to 4 percent prevalence projected by Greenfield, Grant, and Lieberman.[16]

Now it was time to summarize the presentation. Factors contributing to the objectivity of the research project were highlighted. These factors included the use of the preset criteria for hypertension and for obesity, the recording of blood pressure measurements on the backs of the questionnaires before reading the students' responses, and the adoption of a standard critical value for statistical significance before performing any calculations. The accuracy of the interpretations of the research findings was assured by frequent consultation with a statistics professor. The closing sentence before the question-and-answer session addressed the relevancy of this project to community health nursing. The community of high school seniors was identified as the client; community assessment was performed in a research format; community health and prevention of illness were promoted by formal and informal teaching as well as by health screening.

During the frantic rush to clear the stage after the presentation to make room for the next group of students, the group members shared a strong sense of completion. Their project had been well received, but, more importantly, through group effort they had surpassed their own expectations. This celebration was the group's termination.

IMPACT OF THE RESEARCH PROJECT

A summary of the research results was typed and delivered to the school officials in fulfillment of the agreement by which the nursing students had been allowed access to the high schools. Had they been asked at that time, the nursing students would have said that the impact of their study was confined to the individual high school students who participated in the research project.

As time passed, however, the research findings did have a wider impact on the Spokane adolescent community. In the process of developing a grant proposal for the Adolescent Health Center Program, the Spokane County Health

District used the findings of the hypertension research study to document the need for blood pressure screening of adolescents. The Adolescent Health Center Program, which included blood pressure screening in junior and senior high schools among its components, was funded in 1982 by the State of Washington Department of Social and Health Services. The hypertension research study, planned and performed by eight baccalaureate nursing students in two Spokane high schools, thus had an influence on the health of adolescents throughout Spokane county.

CONCLUSION

From the first amorphous planning meeting to the exuberantly orchestrated presentation of the project, these eight community health nursing students learned more than they expected. Completion of the project satisfied a number of the overall course objectives for the community health nursing course. The objectives thus satisfied were

1. Application of the roles of the community nurse as appropriate with the individual family and/or group(s)
2. Use of the nursing process in the provision of health care to provide health care to individuals, families, and/or community (including performing a community assessment project)
3. Initiation of a plan for teaching health concepts to individuals and/or groups in any setting
4. Implementation of a plan for teaching health concepts to individuals and/or groups in any setting
5. Interpretation of trends in nursing and society as they relate to the past, present, and future development of the profession
6. Recognition of the responsibility for continuing education and professional growth.

One of the important functions of the community health nurse is the planning and implementation of community assessment. The students performed this role of the community nurse using a research format. After defining the target community (seniors at two high schools), they identified possible factors that could characterize the population at high risk (for example, positive family history, obesity, and so forth). As they performed the assessment, they also did teaching aimed at promotion of health, another role of the community health nurse. Throughout the process, the community was perceived as the client.

The students' use of the nursing process emphasized the assessment portion of the process. Planning and implementation aspects occurred in the counseling of the high school seniors identified as hypertensive and in the formal and informal health teaching that occurred during the assessment process. The formal teaching sessions also fulfilled the course objectives related to planning and implementation of a teaching plan.

As the nursing students planned the research project, they were cognizant of a societal trend toward learning about one's own body and asking questions about one's own health. They incorporated this "consumer information" trend into the design of their community assessment project. Another trend recognized by the students and incorporated into their choice of assessment format was the increasing importance of research to the nursing profession. Through use of the research format, the students were preparing themselves for the research role of the professional nurse and laying the foundation for continued professional growth in the areas of community assessment and nursing research.

After the presentation, the students thought their project was complete. From choral reading of hypotheses to establishment of an adolescent health program was a step they had not anticipated. Such a beneficial outcome emphasizes the importance of the research approach to community assessment. Through a community assessment project, the students, the community, and the future nursing profession benefitted.

REFERENCES

1. McCALL, RB: *Fundamental Statistics for Psychology.* Harcourt Brace Jovanovich, New York, 1975.

2. AAGAARD, G: *Treatment of hypertension.* In: *Advances in Cardiovascular Nursing.* American Journal of Nursing, New York, 1975.

3. AMERICAN HEART ASSOCIATION: *High Blood Pressure.* American Heart Association, 1969.

4. BATTERMAN, B: *Hypertension, part 1: Detection and evaluation.* Cardio-Vascular Nursing, Vol 11, No 4, July/August 1975, pp 35-40.

5. BERKSON, D AND STANLON J: *The therapy of hypertension. In World Wide Abstracts,* 1965.

6. BIND, RJ: *Alcohol's effects on the heart.* Consultant 14(1):69, 1975.

7. BROWN, AF: *Research in Nursing.* WB Saunders, Philadelphia, 1958.

8. BRUNNER, L AND SUDDARTH, D: *The Lippincott Manual of Nursing Practice.* JB Lippincott, Philadelphia, 1974.

9. BOYER, JL: *What exercise can and cannot do.* Consultant 15(9):110, 1975.

10. GERNIAK AND FEINGOLD: *Birth Control Handbook,* ed 12. 1974.

11. GRITTENDEN, IH: *Hypertension's beginnings. Gleaner,* North Pacific Union Conference, March 7, 1977.

12. FLEMING SW AND HAYTER J: *Reading research reports critically.* Nurs Outlook 22(3):172, 1974.

13. FREIS, ED: *Age, race, sex and other indices of risk in hypertension.* Am J Med 55:275, 1973.

14. GANONG, WF: *Review of Medical Physiology.* Lange Medical Publications, Los Altos, CA, 1969.

15. PELTON, R: *Nicotine and the effects of smoking, and 101 things you should know about marijuana.* In GIRDANO, DD AND GIRDANO, DA: *Drugs: A Factual Account, ed 2.* Addison-Wesley, Reading, MA, 1976.

16. GREENFIELD, D, GRANT, R, LIEBERMAN, E: *Children can have high blood pressure, too.* Am J Nurs 76(5):770, 1976.

17. LANCOUR, J: *How to avoid pitfalls in measuring blood pressure.* Am J Nurs 76(5):773, 1976.

18. LANG, LL, WINSLOW, EH, SCHUEHING, MA, CALLAHAN, JA: *Hypertension: What patients need to know.* Am J Nurs, May 1976, p 766.

19. LUCKMANN, J AND SORENSON, K: *Medical-Surgical Nursing.* WB Saunders, Philadelphia, 1974.

20. MOSER, M: *Epidemiology of primary hypertension with particular reference to racial susceptibility.* In MOYER, J (ED): *Hypertension.* WB Saunders, Philadelphia, 1959.

21. NOTTER, L: *Essentials of Nursing Research.* Springer Publishing, New York, 1974.

22. *Birth Control Handbook.* Planned Parenthood, 1976.

23. SCHROEDER, H: *Hypertension in the Orient.* In MOYER, J (ED): *Hypertension.* WB Saunders, Philadelphia, 1959.

24. SHAFER, KN, SAWYER, JR, McCLUSKEY, AM, BECK, EL, PHIPPS, WJ: *Medical-Surgical Nursing, ed 5.* CV Mosby, St Louis, 1971.

25. SMITH, DW AND GERMAIN, CPH: *Care of the Adult Patient.* JB Lippincott, Philadelphia, 1975.

CHAPTER 15

THE COMMUNITY ASSESSMENT PROJECT

ZANA RAE HIGGS, R.N., Ed.D.

There is a whirl of activity and buzz in the air. Every vacant classroom, nook, and cranny is filled with students making overheads, posters, props; drawing maps; setting up slides; and practicing skits. The communities have been assessed, the presentations are taking form, and the completion and grading of the Community Assessment Projects (CAPs) about to begin. A challenging yet fun break from the usual clinical days of home visits, clinics, agency referrals, and conferences.

The faculty of the Intercollegiate Center for Nursing Education (ICNE) believes that learning how to do a community assessment, like learning to care for individuals and families or understanding group dynamics, requires experiential learning. Each of these areas of knowledge are process focused and, therefore, need to be experienced in order for the content to be applied and for the graduate to be able to perform the activity after graduation.

Therefore, over the last 12 years and in two distinctly different curricular models the community health nursing faculty have required students to perform a community assessment project. Initially CAP was a requirement in the Community Health Nursing course of a medical specialty block curriculum.

During the first workshop week of the course, about 5 hours of content in concepts of community as a client and community assessment with emphasis on Kent's descriptive approach, the epidemiological approach, and Tinkham and Voorhies' assessment tool were provided.[1,2] Following this, each clinical group of between 8 and 10 students chose a community it wished to study. These communities were from a geographic area within Spokane and its surrounding rural county to businesses such as Goodwill Industries, the toll bridge operators, ambulance drivers, and small private industries. Dorms, apartment buildings, public schools, and even the ICNE itself were popular choices.

Once permission was given to pursue the assessment of a specified community, the clinical group was on its own to make the necessary contacts, to organize their time, to delegate tasks, to develop instruments for data collection, and to complete their objectives. Two hours a week of clinical time were allowed in a "to be arranged" format for the students to accomplish this course requirement. The clinical instructor served as a resource, but it was definitely a student project. Students were provided a list of objectives for this learning experience and a copy of the evaluation tool faculty and peers would use to grade their presentation. (See sample instrument and clarifying materials at the end of this chapter.)

Toward the end of the quarter, a full day was set aside from clinical time for student groups to present their CAPs. Each group had 1 hour allotted for its presentation. The presentation could be organized in whatever manner the group felt would best demonstrate accomplishment of the objectives. The faculty and students used the same evaluation tool to grade the presentations.

Each presentation was evaluated immediately after its completion by the audience during a 15-minute break. The evaluation sheets were placed in a large manilla envelope and kept by the clinical instructor. At the end of the day, each clinical group met to review comments on evaluation sheets and to compute their grade. The mean score of peer evaluation was averaged with the mean score of faculty evaluations, and that grade was the CAP grade all group members obtained.

This particular approach required little faculty time other than initiating the process, arranging for classrooms, and serving as resources to students. It required the students to organize, to plan, and to implement a group endeavor; to perform a community assessment; to clearly present their findings, conclusions, and projected planned interventions to their class; and to participate in peer evaluation.

The strengths of this approach are that it allowed students to define a community of interest and to totally organize, arrange and implement their own assessments. It required group endeavor and allowed for application of group process theory to a task group. It provided opportunity for numerous contacts with the community client and allowed for validation of initial impressions and time for provision of feedback to key community members regarding their findings. This might be seen as the initial "unfreezing" step of the change process. It provided students with a structured experience in peer review and allowed for vicarious learning through hearing all clinical group presentations.

The weaknesses of this approach were that it requires students to accomplish this task concurrent with other clinical experiences and that peer evaluation tends to inflate grades. There was no time for implementing with the community the proposed changes or programs. However, implementation was not felt to be a required learning experience for undergraduate students.

When the new curriculum was developed, the community content became a part of a senior year course that required students to expand their concept of client to include groups and communities as well as individuals and families. Group and community concepts are introduced as new content. The content and related learning experience do not focus on high-stress situations. Students perform a CAP and colead a group. In addition, students have clinical experience in assisting individuals and families to cope with high stress, complex health problems in episodic and distributive settings. Weekly group meetings, having regular clinical experiences in an agency, and performing a CAP throughout the term were felt to be activities too fragmenting for students. Therefore, the CAP was organized in the manner described below.

Initial content in a workshop week regarding community as a client, various approaches to community assessment, and sources and types of assessment data are provided. A CAP packet is distributed with the course syllabus. This packet includes worksheets, a community survey, and a CAP presentation evaluation form. (See samples at the end of this chapter.)

During the term, the Community Health Nursing (CHN) faculty members select certain census tracts for clinical groups to assess. Often a census tract is too large for a group to assess in the allotted time, so a representative portion of that tract is identified for assessment purposes.

The CHN faculty members prepare a packet for each clinical group which includes 1) a map of the identified area, 2) raw census tract data for the whole city and the census tract under study, 3) data regarding leading causes of death by age, 4) any community development data the faculty member has been able to obtain, and 5) the name of and appointment time with at least one key informant that the faculty member has provided.

During the last class period prior to the CAP, a faculty member takes approximately 1 hour to prepare the students for the CAP, to pass out the packets, and to allow the students a half hour to meet in clinical groups to review packet materials and to determine how to proceed the following day. The next two days, which are clinical days, are allotted for the students to perform their assessments, to prepare their data for presentation, to determine problems, to identify high-priority problems, and to recommend proposed interventions. Students are expected to start at 8 AM and to proceed to their communities to perform a descriptive assessment using the Kent approach. They are to have delegated among themselves the task of doing house-to-house surveys and of interviewing key informants. That evening each student or group of students collates the data. Each group spends the following morning sharing data, drawing conclusions, and preparing for the presentation.

The afternoon of the second day students present their CAPs. In order to use time efficiently, the student sections and faculty are split into two groups and presentations are made to half the students and faculty simultaneously in two rooms. These are graded using the evaluation tool in the same format previously discussed.

This approach requires more faculty time to develop the packets and to make the arrangements for key informant interviews, as well as to arrange for rooms and to act as resource persons. It requires the students to assess a community using a prepackaged set of tools and approaches. The group must still organize its activities, delegate tasks, collect data, prepare the presentation, and be involved in peer review.

The strengths of this approach are that it allows students to immerse themselves in this learning experience in a short time frame using an eclectic approach to community assessment, it requires a cooperative group endeavor and peer review, and it provides familiarity with a few of the standard approaches to assessment. This approach also is useful for a continuing education workshop.

The major drawback of this format is that it requires the faculty to do much of the preparation and planning of the assessment and does not allow students frequent contact with the community to validate initial impressions and to develop a relationship which can be used to share identified problems and possible solutions.

Another issue in using both evaluation tools is the approximate equal weight they place on assessment and planning. Therefore, if a student is to do a CAP as a part of a challenge examination for a course, the student might do a very superficial job of assessment and still pass the project if the planning phase was strong. However, both approaches have effectively provided students with a learning experience that meets the program objectives and in which students enthusiastically participate.

RATING SCALE FOR EVALUATION OF THE COMMUNITY ASSESSMENT PROJECT

Definitions of Ratings

  0 = Did not cover, objective not met

  6 = Superficial, lacked many essential points, objective met at a minimum level

  7

  8 = Adequately covered, objective met as expected

  9

10 = Thorough, comprehensive coverage, objective met at an excellent level.

Objectives: The group

	0	6	7	8	9	10
ASSESSMENT: Describes the situation thoroughly based on Tinkham and Voorhies' model.						
Gathers pertinent data for identification of problems.						

	0	6	7	8	9	10
Identifies major problems in area.						
Supports problems identified with data collected.						
Assigns priority to the identified health problems giving rationale.						
States limitations of assessment and approaches tried in dealing with limitations.						
Comments						
PLAN: Identifies one main problem and identifies alternative plans of actions in relation to the main problem.						
States preferred plan of action and rationale for the plan.						
States long-range goals to be accomplished by preferred plan.						
Defines measurable outcomes to be accomplished by plan.						
Comments:						
IMPLEMENTATION: Analyzes the relationship of various factors (i.e., political, economic, social, educational, agencies, and resource persons) that might influence the selection of planned implementation.						
Based on the above factors, identifies ideal and realistic approaches, selecting the one best method of implementation.						

	0	6	7	8	9	10
Identifies and prioritizes specific implementation steps.						
Comments:						
EVALUATION OF IMPLEMENTATION: Describes the method of approach to evaluation proposed.						
States the strengths of the method of evaluation.						
States the weaknesses of the method of evaluation.						
Comments:						
For the presentation process, evaluate the group (0) objective not met, (6) objective met at minimal level, (8) objective met as expected, (10) objective met at an excellent level.						
PRESENTATION PROCESS:						
Functions smoothly and cohesively as a group during the presentation.						
Elicits the interest of the viewer by methods of presentation (creativity).						
Presents material in an organized manner (uses time effectively).						
Manages questions and answer period(s) effectively.						
Comments:						

Rater's Total Score _____

From N440, Community Health Nursing, Intercollegiate Center for Nursing Education.

CASE STUDIES IN COMMUNITY ASSESSMENT

CLARIFICATION OF RATING SCALE FOR EVALUATION OF THE COMMUNITY ASSESSMENT PROJECT

The following are additional comments related to the objectives to be met by students' CAP.

ASSESSMENT:
1. Describes the situation thoroughly based on Tinkham and Voorhies' model.
   Refers to breadth and depth of thoroughness of assessment and ability to utilize and organize data using the assigned model.
2. Gathers pertinent data for identification of problems.
   Is there sufficient data to allow for problem identification and prioritization?
3. Identifies major problems in area.
   Definition of needs/nursing diagnoses.
4. Supports problems identified with data collected.
   Can these problems be supported by the data collected?
5. Assigns priority to the identified health problems giving rationale.
   What forms the basis for priorities (e.g., the nature of the problems, the political/social expediency based on community motivation, and so forth)?
6. States limitations of assessment and approaches tried in dealing with limitations.
   Clearly identify what data you feel were important but did not collect and why they were not collected. How reliable is the information collected? How did you try to deal with limitations/barriers?

PLAN:
7. Identifies one main problem and identifies alternative plans of action in relation to the main problem.
   Based on #5 above, select your top priority problems. Identify alternative actions which you and the community might take to solve the problem.
8. States the preferred plan of action and rationale for the plan.
   Why did you choose the alternative you selected?
9. States the long-range goals to be accomplished by the preferred plan.
   What change do you wish to occur?
10. Defines measurable outcomes to be accomplished by the plan.
    These are the statements of measurable outcome criteria against which you will judge the effectiveness of your interventions.

IMPLEMENTATION:
11. Analyzes the relationships of various factors (i.e., political, economic, social, educational, agencies, and resource persons) that might influence the selection of planned implementation.
    Use what you know about change theory in your analysis.
12. Based on the above factors, identifies ideal and realistic approaches, selecting the one best method of implementation.

Identify what you would do under ideal circumstances (no limitations of money, manpower, material, and motivation). What can realistically be done, given the constraints of the situation?
13. Identifies and prioritizes *specific* implementation *steps.*
Write out step by step the approach you would take to accomplish your outcomes noted in #10.

EVALUATION:
14. Describes the method/approach to evaluation proposed.
How do you plan to evaluate? What tool(s) will you use? What data will you collect?
15. States the strengths of the method of evaluation.
This includes your rationale for selection of evaluation method/approach.
16. States the weakness of the method of evaluation.
What are the limitations of this method/approach?

PRESENTATION PROCESS:
17. Functions smoothly and cohesively as a group during presentation.
Audience informed regarding group's plan for presentation and role of members therein. Demonstrated through interchanges among group members during presentation.
18. Elicits the interest of the viewer by methods of presentation.
Creative, varies stimuli (see Teaching/Learning Process Packet).
19. Presents material in organized manner.
Audience should be able to readily obtain information for objectives #1 through 16. Presentation should flow smoothly and interrelatedness of the whole process should be clear.
20. Manages question and answer period(s) effectively.
Provides for question. Acknowledges audience need for additional clarification and provides it.

From N440, Community Health Nursing, Intercollegiate Center for Nursing Education.

COMMUNITY ASSESSMENT PROJECT WORKSHEET

OUTLINE	NOTES
ASSESSMENT	
I. Descriptive Approach	
A. Physical	
1. Space defined	
2. Boundaries	
3. Barriers	
a. Geographic	
b. Access	
c. Traffic	

         d. Fences
      4. Patterns of movement
      5. Signs
      6. Transportation
      7. Structures (churches, schools, homes, business)
      8. Recreational facilities
   B. Social (management of environment)
      1. Orientation
         a. Labor
         b. Religion
         c. Rural/urban
         d. Time
      2. Gathering places
      3. Helping systems
         a. Caretaker/natural helper
         b. Communication
            1) Communicators
            2) Networks
            3) Formal/informal
      4. Play
   C. Economics
      1. Work
      2. Health care
      3. Financial controls
      4. Government assistance
      5. Handling money
         a. Food stamps
         b. Check cashing
         c. Purchasing
   D. Concluding themes
II. Statistical
   A. Demographic data
   B. Concluding themes
III. Interview data
   A. Key informants
      1. Interviewing the key informants:
         Key informants are individuals within a community who are in a position of formal or informal power and influence or at the center of a communications network. These people usually have a finger on the pulse of the community. Therefore, they have a perspective on the health problems and concerns of the community. They also know the community's way of functioning, who the key leaders are that influence decisions in the community, what are the community's resources, and what the decision-making process is in the community. These are important considerations in planning your proposed

---

THE COMMUNITY ASSESSMENT PROJECT   **175** project. We have tried to identify at least one person in each community who can provide you with this perspective. Remember, it is this person's view and may not be objective. So in compiling your data you need to look for common themes among all sources.

    B. Concluding themes
    C. Survey (see attached)
    D. Concluding themes
 IV. Problems identified
    (problem list)

PLANNING/PROPOSED PROJECT
   I. Selected problem/rationale
  II. Proposed project
 III. Proposed evaluation

From N406, Clinical Nursing III, Intercollegiate Center for Nursing Education. Spacing has been condensed for publication.

COMMUNITY ASSESSMENT PROJECT SURVEY

Interview Schedule

I am a student nurse at the Intercollegiate Center for Nursing Education. As a part of our program we are involved in assessing the health needs of a community. I have been assigned to assess the health needs of this area. We would like to know what concerns people who live in the community have about health, so my fellow students and I are doing a door-to-door survey of opinions of people in the neighborhood. We will summarize all the opinions and share the survey with our fellow students and instructors.

Would you be willing to answer a few questions about the degree to which different health problems are of concern in this community?

I will read you a list of health problems. Please tell me if it is a major problem for people who live in this community, if it is somewhat of a problem, or if you think it is not a problem in this community.

Potential Health Problems	Major problem 2	Somewhat of a problem 1	Not a problem 0	Notes
Contagious childhood disease (measles, mumps, chickenpox)				
Children not immunized				
Child neglect or abuse				

Potential Health Problems	Major problem 2	Somewhat of a problem 1	Not a problem 0	Notes
Juvenile delinquency (vandalism/truancy)				
Emotional problems in children				
Scabies, lice, ringworm				
Malnutrition (poor/inadequate diet)				
Overweight/obesity				
Arthritis; rheumatism				
Upper respiratory tract infections (colds or flu)				
Chronic lung problems (emphysema)				
High blood pressure (hypertension)				
Accidents/injuries				
Heart conditions other than stroke (heart attack, heart problems requiring medication)				
Stroke (CVA)				
Tuberculosis (TB)				
Venereal/sexually transmitted disease (syphilis/gonorrhea/herpes)				
Cancer				
Physical disability that limits work/activity				
Mental disability that limits work/activity				
Loneliness (few friends and social contacts)				
Tension/stress				
Depression				
Suicide/attempted suicide				
Alcoholism or drinking problem				

Potential Health Problems	Major problem 2	Somewhat of a problem 1	Not a problem 0	Notes
Problems with drugs or drug abuse other than alcohol (marijuana)				
Family/marital conflict				
Pregnancy in young teenagers				
Crimes against persons (assault, rape, murder)				
Crimes against property (burglary, vandalism)				
Unemployment				
Low income/financial distress				
Unsafe to go out in neighborhood				
Air pollution				
Noise				
Litter/trash (dogs, cats, rodents)				
Lack of community spirit				

Now I would like to ask you to what degree are the following agencies or services a problem in the community. Please answer if the service is adequate, inadequate, or nonexistent.

Agency/Service	Nonexistent 2	Inadequate 1	Adequate 0	Notes
Water				
Garbage collection/service				
Police				
Schools				
Day care facilities				
Hospital or emergency care facilities				
Doctor's offices/clinics				
Prenatal/well-child care services				

Agency/Service	Nonexistent 2	Inadequate 1	Adequate 0	Notes
Mental health services				
Crisis intervention services				
Churches				
Social organizations				
Restaurants				
Grocery stores				
Postal service				
Communication (radio/tv/newspaper)				
General shopping facilities				
Public transportation				
Access to government officials				
Traffic control				
Gas/electricity service				
Telephone service				

What do you believe is the most important health concern for this community?

What would you like to see done about it?

How are you using community resources?

Thank you for helping us by participating in this survey.
                    Students of the Intercollegiate Center for Nursing Education

From N406, Clinical Nursing III, Intercollegiate Center for Nursing Education.

CURRENT RATING SCALE FOR EVALUATION OF COMMUNITY ASSESSMENT PROJECT

Rating Consideration

Rating should be determined on the basis of thoroughness of information, objectivity, and clarity with which it is presented and degree to which data support conclusions made. *Please make comments clarifying ratings after each item.*

95% Outstanding Performance: Students consistently met objectives at a high level. Information was thorough and comprehensive; well organized and clearly presented within time allowed. Integration of theoretical concepts in analysis of data and planned interventions was excellent. Data were strongly supportive of conclusions.

85% Above Average Performance: Students consistently met objectives. Information, although present, occasionally lacked organization or clarity of presentation. Level lacked depth. Analysis of data and planned interventions demonstrated integration of theoretical concepts. Data supported conclusions.

75% Average Performance: Objectives were met with occasional gaps of information. At times presentation was difficult to follow or it was difficult to determine major points. Application of theoretical concepts was inconsistent. Relationships between data and conclusions were sometimes unclear.

65% Below Average: Objectives were not met. Major portions of information were missing. There was a lack of clarity in presentation and/or limited application of theoretical concepts. Conclusions were generally not supported by data.

0% Unacceptable: Objectives were not met. Information was absent.

	0	65	75	85	95
ASSESSMENT 1. Describe the community based on Kent's approach.					
2. Describe the community based on demographic data.					
3. Describe the health concerns identified by key informant(s).					
4. Describe the health concerns identified in the survey.					
5. State the limitations of the overall assessment.					
6. Identify resources that could be used to obtain supplemental data in relation to #5.					
7. Identify problems/health needs within the community (Problem list).					
8. Data collected support problems identified.					

	0	65	75	85	95
PLAN/PROPOSED PROJECTS 1. Provide rationale for categorizing health problems in terms of priority and for the selection of the problem chosen for intervention.					
2. Identify method you would use to validate your conclusions in #1.					
3. Identify long-range goals and measurable outcomes to be accomplished by the project.					
4. Describe proposed project.					
5. Identify factors within the community that should be considered in initiating the project (e.g., key community issues, beliefs, power sources, political, social, economic, educational, existing agencies and resources.)					
6. Based on the above factors, identify both ideal and realistic approaches, selecting the one best method of implementation.					
7. Identify steps you would take to initiate the project.					
8. Explain the method/approach you plan to use to determine the success of the project.					

Score _____

From N406, Clinical Nursing III, Intercollegiate Center for Nursing Education. Spacing has been condensed for publication.

REFERENCES

1. KENT, J: *A descriptive approach to community*. In: *Five Years of Cooperation to Improve Curriculum in Western Schools of Nursing*. Western Interstate Commission for Higher Education, Boulder, CO, March 1972.

2. TINKHAM, C AND VOORHIES, E: *Community Health Nursing: Evaluation and Process*. Appleton-Century-Crofts, New York, 1977, pp 277–290.

APPLICATION OF NURSING THEORIES

One of the evolutionary directions for nursing as a profession has been to define nursing and the activities nursing encompasses. General definitions and standards have been developed to serve as guides for all those who practice nursing. An outcome of this process has been the development of models and theories of nursing. Just as individual nurses may practice in their own unique styles while adhering to the guidelines developed by their profession, each model or theory uses a particular vocabulary, definition of philosophy, and conceptual focus as a framework to assist the nurse in providing care to the client with a health disorder.

No particular model or theory has been judged superior to another. A few models are being used as the conceptual basis for curricula in schools of nursing. Others are serving as the basis for practice in episodic agencies. Most have been designed to guide nursing care for the individual client. The purpose of this unit is not to establish the efficacy of any particular model or theory but to present selected approaches to demonstrate their applicability to assessment of the community as a client.

We wish to thank LaVonne Berentson, Sheila Masteller, Edith Coleman, Sherri Howard, and Carol Allen who so graciously contributed their ideas to the following selections.

183

CHAPTER 16

THE OREM MODEL APPLIED TO COMMUNITY ASSESSMENT*

LaVONNE BERENTSON, R.N., M.S.N.

Conceptual models are useful in nursing as frameworks to organize and to provide the focus for the content of nursing. These frameworks suggest theories to be tested, organize the borrowing and/or adapting of relevant theories from other disciplines, and give direction for research. A model's usefulness is to be judged by the amount of theoretical material it organizes and the testable theories it generates.

Newman suggests the following relationships of models to nursing theories.[1] The conceptual framework or model suggests the focus of inquiry. From the framework, concepts are identified and assumptions about the field of inquiry are articulated. These concepts then suggest relationships among themselves, providing testable theories.

Conceptual Framework (Model)
↓
Identifying Concepts
↓
Theories Relating the Concepts to Each Other
↓
Research

*The ideas presented in this chapter were developed while I was teaching in the RN-BSN program at Lewis-Clark State College, Lewiston, Idaho. I wish to thank Marion Leech, RN, BSN; Tricia Tate, RN, BSN; and Brian Fonnesbeck, RN, BSN; who assisted in the development of the format for the Community Assessment Tool and allowed me to incorporate many of their ideas into this chapter. I especially want to thank Paula Herberg, RN, MS, teaching colleague, with whom many hours were spent debating the constructs of the Orem model.

Conceptual frameworks applied to the assessment and care of the community as a client can help nursing develop its own unique community health knowledge base. They can assist with the blending of knowledge from sociology, public health, and nursing to make a unique entity. They can also suggest research that will help build the nursing knowledge base.

COMMUNITY THEORY AND OREM'S MODEL FOR NURSING PRACTICE

In this chapter I have combined some of the work of community theorists with the Orem model for nursing practice. It is by no means exhaustive, but it is a beginning attempt to organize community theory into a framework that can be helpful to nurses viewing the community as a client.

The usefulness of a nursing model and community theory to nursing practice can be determined by nurses using it in their daily practice. It is through this process that nurses can choose those elements which are helpful and research new elements suggested by the use of models and their theoretical components.

The concepts of the Orem model that are pertinent to the assessment and diagnosis of a community's health self-care status are 1) universal self-care requisites, 2) developmental self-care requisites, 3) health-deviation self-care requisites, 4) therapeutic self-care demand, 5) self-care agency, 6) self-care deficits, and 7) adequate self-care actions.[2] The concepts of universal, developmental, and health-deviation self-care requisites and therapeutic self-care demand are theoretical constructs which provide guidelines to determine the data that are needed for the assessment of the community self-care agency. The information in each of these areas comes from community theorists and community research. It is the knowledge base that is used by the nurse to assess the community as a client.

The model is based on the assumption that all clients have the right to and responsibility of their own self-care. The area of self-care that is of primary interest to the nurse is self-care relative to health concerns. However, because all the subsystems within the community client system are interrelated, the action of one subsystem affects all the other subsystems. Therefore, all community subsystems need to be assessed to learn both how they impinge on health-related self-care functioning and where in the system intervention efforts are most likely to be successful.

Before Orem's model to community assessment is applied, it is necessary to define concepts of Orem's model in relation to the community. There are three categories of requisites: universal self-care requisites, developmental self-care requisites, and health-deviation self-care requisites. Requisites are defined as that which is required or necessary for some purpose.[3] All communities share universal and developmental self-care requisites. Universal requisites are those needs common to all communities; regardless of the size, location, or degree of modernization. Developmental self-care requisites arise from the universal self-care requisites and are those needs associated with the process of change and development of a community. These developmental requisites deal with a community's need to continue to provide for the fulfillments of its universal self-care requisites as conditions change either within or outside the community system. Health-deviation self-care requisites are needs associated with dysfunction within the community. They arise when a community is experiencing threats to its well being.

The term self-care agency is used to depict the ability of a community to evaluate and to perform the functions necessary to maintain its self-care. When a community is adequately meeting its self-care requisites, there is no need for nursing intervention.

Therapeutic self-care demands are the actions that a community must take to maintain its present level of functioning or to move toward more desirable levels of functioning. If the demand related to health care is greater than the ability of the community's self-care agency, then a self-care deficit exists and the need for the nursing agency is introduced.

Nursing agency is the ability of the nurse to provide for the maintenance, health, and well being of the community with health-related self-care deficits. It must be noted here that the nurse is functioning within the community in dual capacities. When the community is viewed as the client, the nurse is the assessor and intervenor in the event of a self-care deficit. The nurse also functions as a part of the community's self-care agency. If the requisites of the community are met while the nurse is functioning in a usual capacity, a self-care deficit does not exist. If the usual activities within the system do not meet the therapeutic self-care demands, the nursing agency will be required to meet the self-care deficit.

The nursing agency uses the nursing process to observe the community, to analyze its problems, and to assist it through the basic nursing systems. The functions a professional performs to assist the client are classified into five methods: acting for and doing for another, support, guiding, providing a developmental environment, and teaching. There are three basic nursing systems: wholly compensatory, partly compensatory, and supportive-educative. When the client is an individual, the wholly compensatory system requires the nurse to perform the total care of the client. This would be a rare situation for a community client. An example could be a flood that devastates an entire community. For a time, the total community may be unable to function. Because it is a community client, the need for total assistance from outside the community would involve an interdisciplinary team effort. The partly compensatory system requires both the nurse and the client to provide parts of the care needed. In the supportive-educative system, the client is able to perform most of its own self-care but needs support and education from the nurse.

The ultimate goal is that the client achieve or regain a self-care agency that can maintain adequate self-care action. When the total self-care is not feasible, the goal is to maintain the greatest amount of self-care with the least assistance from the nurse that is possible. The self-care agency of the client community is the entity that is to be assessed.

The concepts of self-care deficits and adequate self-care actions are the di-

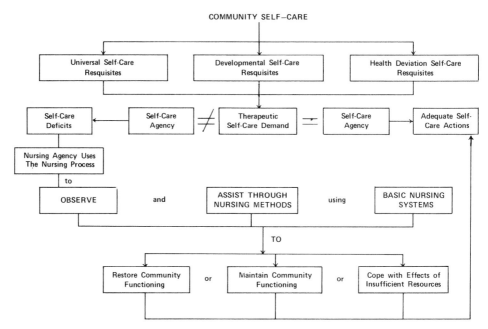

FIGURE 16-1. Schematic representation of community self-care.

agnostic constructs. The ability of the community's self-care agency to meet its therapeutic self-care demands determines whether it has a self-care deficit related to particular therapeutic self-care demands or if it has adequate self-care actions related to those particular self-care demands (Fig. 16-1).

UNIVERSAL SELF-CARE REQUISITES

Klein,[4] a community theorist, writes about the community in relation to mental health activities. His concepts can be expanded to encompass all of community health self-care. The assumption that the community is responsible for the health and well being of its members underlies the universal self-care requisites.

According to Klein,[5] the community needs to be more than the setting in which the mental health agency resides but must instead be the essential source of mental health itself. This idea can be expanded to see the community as the source of the physical and mental well being of its individual members and not solely as the repository of the services for dealing with illness and disease.

The community imposes the condition of living on its members. This means that the value a community holds for a particular person is going to determine to a large extent that person's health status.[6] For example, a valued member of the community will have a greater use of space, goods, and services available than a person deemed less valuable. Therefore, an owner of a community business will have access to better food, medical services, perhaps superior sanitation and cleaner air than a person on welfare. When individuals receive less than an adequate share of the goods and services that lead to general well being, the basic assumption underlying the universal self-care requisites is violated. This could impinge on their health status.

Collectively, the universal self-care requisites of a community are to provide adequately for all members of the community. Klein's major functions of a community are used here as the universal self-care requisites for a community. They are

1. Providing and distributing living space and shelter and determining use of space for other purposes;
2. Making available the means for distributing necessary goods and services;
3. Maintaining safety and order, and facilitating the resolution of conflicts;
4. Educating and acculturating newcomers (e.g., children and immigrants);
5. Transmitting information, ideas, and beliefs;
6. Creating and enforcing rules and standards of belief and behavior;
7. Providing opportunities for interaction between individuals and groups.[7]

THERAPEUTIC SELF-CARE DEMANDS FOR UNIVERSAL SELF-CARE REQUISITES

Therapeutic self-care demands are the actions that a community must take to meet the self-care requisites of a community. The demands related to universal self-care requisites are that the community provide

1. a. The planning and zoning of land;
   b. Adequate housing, parks, and recreational areas;
   c. Industrial and agricultural areas.
2. a. Business areas providing the necessary goods and services;
   b. Goods and services that are readily accessible to community residents;
   c. Adequate health service facilities and personnel;
   d. An adequate economic base;
   e. Adequate numbers of professional and service people;
   f. Public assistance.
3. a. Police and fire service;
   b. Public health measures, the setting and enforcement of environmental standards, e.g., sewer, water, air pollution;
   c. Governmental forms to handle special interests and the conflicts of interest;

d. Courts and the legal system.
4. a. Schools (preschool through high school, access to post-secondary education, vocational education, and continuing education);
   b. Sufficient openness and mobility into community groups.
5. a. Mass media;
   b. Churches;
   c. Civic, social, and academic organizations.
6. a. Community ordinances;
   b. Community norms.
7. a. Community forums, e.g., town meetings, letters to the editor.

DEVELOPMENTAL SELF-CARE REQUISITES

Community development is used in this model to depict the need of the community to change as resources, shifting population patterns, and altered ecology change the nature of the universal self-care requisites. For example, an increasingly commercialized small town may need to change zoning ordinances to redistribute the space between business/industry and residential areas.

The theoretical material for community development is taken from Edwards and Jones.[8] They describe community development as a process. It is the means whereby the people in a community unite to promote what they consider to be necessary for the well being of the community. Some change is undirected and some is directed by individuals or groups with special interests. Other changes are made by the people of the community working together toward common goals.

The persons within a community who decide to make a change proceed from a value orientation that they can and should make or block a change. Once a community action is started by some element within the community, the community uses the networks and linkages among individuals and groups already present in the community. The linkages are a network of roles and statuses. These exist as various informal and formal groups throughout the community's social structure. These linkages, together with other demographic and ecological features of the community, determine the setting from which a need arose, the resources available, and the obstacles to that action that may arise. These community actions represent the community development process.

Community actions are composed of two interrelated aspects. These are the problem-solving activities engaged in by the community to achieve a goal and the effects of these problem-solving activities on the people's ability to continue to work together to develop their community.

As people in a community work together, they may gain positive values, attitudes, and ways of thinking that are as important as their material achievements. These are important because they will facilitate meeting the needs that continue to arise within a community.

TABLE 16-1. Universal Self-Care Requisites and the Corresponding Developmental Self-Care Requisites

UNIVERSAL SELF-CARE REQUISITES*	DEVELOPMENTAL SELF-CARE REQUISITES
1. Providing and distributing living space and shelter and determining use of space for other purposes;	1. Providing the mechanisms to meet the changing needs of space for living, shelter, and other purposes;
2. Making available the means for distribution of necessary goods and services;	2. Providing the mechanisms to meet the changing patterns of consumption of goods and services;
3. Maintaining safety and order and facilitating the resolution of conflicts;	3. Providing the mechanisms to maintain safety with changing patterns of crime, environmental hazards, and community conflicts;
4. Educating and acculturating newcomers (e.g., children and adults);	4. Providing the mechanisms to meet the changing information and socialization needs of children and adults in the community and newcomers with a variety of cultural/educational backgrounds;
5. Transmitting information, ideas, and beliefs;	5. Providing mechanisms for the changing needs of the community for information, ideas, and beliefs;
6. Creating and enforcing rules and standards of belief and behavior;	6. Providing the mechanisms for creating and enforcing new rules for changing patterns of belief and behavior;
7. Providing opportunities for interaction between individuals and groups.	7. Providing the mechanisms for the changing needs for interaction between individuals and groups.

*Community functions according to Klein.[4]

The more separated a community is into different racial, ethnic, income, social class, and life style groups, the more difficult it will be to work together collectively for social action. The ability to work together is facilitated by finding the common values and goals of the different groups.

This community development theory gives the theoretical content for the developmental self-care requisites within the Orem framework. Developmental self-care requisites arise out of the universal self-care requisites. They become evident as the community or element(s) within the community feel the need for a change.

DEVELOPMENTAL THERAPEUTIC SELF-CARE REQUISITES

The self-care actions responding to the therapeutic self-care demands for developmental self-care requisites are elements that Edwards and Jones[9] state are necessary for the process of community development. Each of these elements is necessary for the meeting of any one of the developmental self-care requisites. For example, the same elements are necessary to provide the mechanism for the changing needs of space for living, shelter, and other purposes as to provide the mechanisms to meet the changing patterns of goods and services. The therapeutic self-care demands for each developmental self-care requisite are

1. Involvement of the people within the community in efforts to reach common goals;
2. An emotional commitment by the people of the community to common goals;
3. An articulation of the community's goals;
4. Designing of procedures to attain goals;
5. Attention to the felt needs of the people of the community for a change;
6. Attention given to the sociocultural, demographic, and ecological features of the community as a whole.[10]

Table 16-1 lists the universal self-care requisites and the developmental self-care requisites arising from them.

HEALTH-DEVIATION SELF-CARE REQUISITES

Unlike universal self-care requisites or developmental self-care requisites, health-deviation self-care requisites are not necessarily present within the community. They arise when the community's well being is threatened.

Health deviations that may exist within the community are such problems as crime; poverty, environmental pollution; a natural disaster, such as a flood or

---

tornado; epidemics of communicable diseases, such as measles or hepatitis; and noncontagious diseases, such as emphysema or coronary disease.

Health-deviation self-care requisites are precipitated when a health-deviation exists. The health-deviation self-care requisites are a modification of Orem's health-deviation self-care requisites for individuals.[11] The community must

1. Recognize a threat to the community's well-being,
2. Apply a remedy to seek help for the problem,
3. Implement measures to alleviate the threat.

The following are the therapeutic self-care demands (actions) necessitated by the health-deviation self-care requisites. The community must provide

1. Mechanisms to monitor the state of community functioning and must detect any threat to its well-being;
2. Problem-solving mechanisms within the community and access to external resources;
3. Resources necessary to implement a plan to alleviate the problem.

COMMUNITY SELF-CARE AGENCY

The self-care agency of the community is the entity to be assessed by the nurse. The self-care requisites and their accompanying therapeutic self-care demands provide the theoretical content needed to guide the assessment.

The following example illustrates how the nurse can use these theoretical concepts to determine the data that need to be obtained. One universal self-care requisite is the provision and distribution of living space and shelter and determining use of space for other purposes. A therapeutic self-care demand growing out of that requisite is that the community provide for adequate housing, parks, and recreational areas. The nurse now has theoretical concepts to guide the assessment, such as determining the number of housing units, the number of people per unit; sanitation facilities and utilities available; density of housing; number of people per park; proximity of parks to people; available recreational facilities; the financial ability of people to use the facilities, and so forth.

SELF-CARE DEFICITS AND ADEQUATE SELF-CARE ACTIONS

Self-care deficit and adequate self-care action are the diagnostic concepts within the model. When the community self-care agency is assessed, it can be determined if it is equal to or not equal to the therapeutic self-care demands necessitated by each of the self-care requisites. The diagnosis is then either adequate self-care action related to a specific situation or self-care deficit related to a specific situation.

An illustration may help clarify this concept. An area in a community has a contaminated water supply. This health deviation precipitates health-deviation self-care requisites. To assess the self-care agency of the community, it is then necessary to determine if it is capable of meeting the therapeutic self-care demands. This involves asking the following questions: 1) Is the community monitoring for contaminated water supply? 2) Does the community possess the resources to determine how to correct the situation or how to get help from outside the community if it is unable to solve the problem itself? 3) Does it have the resources, people, time, money, motivation, and so forth to remedy the problem? If the self-care agency cannot meet the therapeutic self-care demand for some reason, such as being unwilling to spend money in that area of the community, the diagnosis would be "Self-care deficit related to lack of motivation to provide healthy water supply."

ASSESSMENT TOOL

An extensive assessment tool can be devised from the theoretical concepts. A tool that is based on theoretical content about the community can assist the nurse to view the whole community system and its relationship to its supersystem and subsystems. It will also help nurses from becoming so absorbed in their own subsystem that they fail to see the whole system.

A detailed, elaborate tool may be useful at certain times, such as when there is a major health problem or when an extensive new approach to a health-care problem is being planned. Portions of the tool may be useful for smaller or more routine problems or projects.

The usefulness of any tool can be determined only by nurses using it in their professional practice. This process will lead to the refinement of a tool as the useful categories are retained and the unnecessary ones eliminated. The use of the tool should also suggest areas in which research is needed to develop the theoretical knowledge base of community health nursing. Table 16-2 is an example of a community assessment tool using Orem's model.

CONCLUSION

A complete tool would list all the self-care requisites and the corresponding therapeutic self-care demands. In the example, space is provided to record the data about the self-care agency that is necessary to determine the self-care agency's ability to meet the therapeutic self-care demands. The sample tool has hypothetical data supplied for a self-care requisite from each of the three self-care requisite areas. The tool illustrates how the theoretical constructs guide the assessment process and lead to community diagnoses.

TABLE 16-2. Community Assessment Tool Using Orem's Model

A. UNIVERSAL SELF-CARE REQUISITES

UNIVERSAL SELF-CARE REQUISITES	THERAPEUTIC SELF-CARE DEMAND	SELF-CARE AGENCY (DATA)	ADEQUATE SELF-CARE ACTIONS OR SELF-CARE DEFICITS
Providing and distributing living space and shelter and determining use of space for other purposes.	The community provides 1. Planning and zoning of land 2. Adequate housing, parks, and recreational areas.	The city, Erehwon, is zoned into business, industrial, and residential areas. The industrial area is separated from the residential and business areas. Heavy equipment, noise, and so forth, do not affect the other two areas. Business areas are close to residential areas, but zoning ordinances prevent both areas from encroaching on each other. There is one centrally located 2-acre city park for 100,000 people. There are 70,000 housing units in the city. The price of homes range from $30,000 to $150,000;	Adequate self-care action related to zoning of business, industrial, and residential areas. Adequate self-care action related to housing and recreational facilities. Self-care deficit related to planning and zoning for parks.

TABLE 16-2. Community Assessment Tool Using Orem's Model—continued

A. UNIVERSAL SELF-CARE REQUISITES

UNIVERSAL SELF-CARE REQUISITES	THERAPEUTIC SELF-CARE DEMAND	SELF-CARE AGENCY (DATA)	ADEQUATE SELF-CARE ACTIONS OR SELF-CARE DEFICITS
		houses rent from $165-600/month, and apartments rent for $150-400/month. There are four low-income subsidized housing developments. There is usually a short waiting list for these units. Commercial recreational facilities are located in each residential area.	

B. DEVELOPMENTAL SELF-CARE REQUISITES

DEVELOPMENTAL SELF-CARE REQUISITES	THERAPEUTIC SELF-CARE DEMAND	SELF-CARE AGENCY (DATA)	ADEQUATE SELF-CARE ACTIONS OR SELF-CARE DEFICITS
Providing the mechanisms to meet the changing needs of	1. Involvement of the people within the community in effort to	Erehwon has a Planning Commission and Board of Adjustment which	Adequate self-care action concerning the self-care deficit related to zoning

space for living, shelter, and other purposes.

reach common goals.
2. An emotional commitment by the people.
3. An articulation of the community's goals.
4. Designing of procedures to attain goal.
5. Attention to the felt need of the people of the community for a change.
6. Attention given to the sociocultural, demographic, and ecological features of the community as a whole.

meets twice a month. They are in charge of the planning and zoning of the land. Regarding the self-care deficit related to planning and zoning for parks: There have been large representations from the community at Planning Commission meeting to protest the lack of parks. The Commission in response to these protests has formulated a plan to zone for and purchase the necessary land for the parks. Attention is being given to forming committees representing the different sociocultural and demographic areas of the community to choose the park areas that would best meet their needs.

and planning for parks.

TABLE 16-2. Community Assessment Tool Using Orem's Model—*continued*

C. HEALTH-DEVIATION SELF-CARE REQUISITES

HEALTH DEVIATION SELF-CARE REQUISITES	THERAPEUTIC SELF-CARE DEMANDS	SELF-CARE AGENCY (DATA)	ADEQUATE SELF-CARE ACTIONS OR SELF-CARE DEFICITS
1. Recognize a threat to the community's well being.	1. Mechanisms to monitor the state of community functioning and to detect any threat to its well being.	Public health department functions to gather data about the incidence of measles. School, private physicians report the incidence of the disease to the department. Health department analyze data to determine existence of an epidemic. The public health department is mounting a campaign to educate the public about the disease, the care of the person with the disease, and an immunization program. The public health department has the public	Adequate self-care action related to measles epidemic.
2. Apply a remedy or seek help for the problem.	2. Problem-solving mechanism within the community access to external resources.		
3. Implement measures to alleviate the threat.	3. Resources necessary to implement a plan to alleviate the problem.		

health nurse see children in the schools, talk to PTAs, and conduct immunization clinics. The schools are distributing information to the children to take home. The local media are covering the epidemic with stories and information.

REFERENCES

1. NEUMAN, M: *Theory Development in Nursing*. FA Davis, Philadelphia, 1979, p 13.

2. OREM, DE: *Nursing: Concepts of Practice*, ed 2. McGraw-Hill, New York, 1980.

3. *Webster's New World Dictionary*, college ed 2. William Collins, Cleveland, 1979.

4. KLEIN, DC: *Community Dynamics and Mental Health*. John Wiley & Sons, New York, 1968.

5. Ibid, p viii.

6. Ibid, p 6.

7. Ibid, p 7.

8. EDWARDS, AD AND JONES, DG: *Community and Community Development*. Mauton, The Hague, Netherlands, 1976.

9. Ibid.

10. Ibid, p 139.

11. OREM, op. cit, pp 50-51.

CHAPTER 17

ASSESSMENT OF A GLEANING COMMUNITY

SHEILA L. MASTELLER, R.N., M.S.
EDITH P. COLEMAN, R.N., M.S.

A community health nursing model revised from the Betty Neuman Care System Model and the Orem Self-Care Concept was developed and used to assess the health needs of the gleaning community in a northwestern metropolitan area.

Gleaning is the gathering and sharing of food after the commercial harvest is completed. Gleaning programs are self-help programs in which low-income people work to help themselves meet their food needs. Mead[1] describes the fairly simple design of the programs. Growers donate produce that is left after the commercial harvest. The food is picked by low-income people gleaning for themselves, and excess is shared with senior citizens, handicapped persons, shelter homes, and meal sites.

A lead organization, such as a community action organization, coordinates each gleaning project. Volunteers in the community work with the lead organization to recruit growers into the program, to organize teams, to arrange transportation to the field, to assist with food preservation and distribution, and to promote the project to others in the community.

Gleaning projects involve gleaners directly in the operation, planning, and growth of their project organizations. Participants in this gleaning project included the field pickers, team or field bosses, project directors, and advisory board members. Gleaning projects not only provide the opportunity for low-income people to help themselves while helping others but also foster community involvement.

CONCEPTUAL MODEL

The community health nursing model we developed is a systems model and has three major components: community, health, community health nursing. These components are a system that exists within a greater system. Self-care is a significant aspect of all three of these components and can be defined as the activities that people "initiate and perform on their own behalf to maintain life, health and well-being."[2]

The Neuman model which presents the individual as the focus of nursing has been modified by replacing the individual with the community as the focus of community health nursing. According to Williams,[3] community health nurses promote community health by concerning themselves with aggregates or population groups.

The diagrammatic representation of our model is shown in Figure 17-1. This model considers the open community system in interaction with its environment, its components of population, environment and resources, the occurrence of stressors to the community system, the reaction of the community system to stressors, the output or health state of the community, and the nursing interactions with the community.

Population, environment, and resources are the community structural elements derived from the model by Clemen, Eigsti, and McGuire.[4] The population is a consciously identified aggregate with demographic, biological, and psycho-social-cultural components. Environment is the society within which the population exists with physical, biochemical, and social components. Resources are the service systems available to the community to promote and to maintain its state of health. Resource components are organizational services and the health care system services.

The dynamic composite of the interrelationships of the three components makes each community unique and affects the community's ability to respond to stressors and, by determining the effect of stressors on the community system, determines the health state of the community.

Communities are subject to many intracommunity, intercommunity, and extracommunity stressors, and each individual community responds uniquely to stressors. Additionally, each community has its own perception of its stressors and its health state. Community health nurses consider the community's perceptions as they collaborate with the community to promote its health.

Health is a dynamic relative state of well being and is illustrated on the model as the jagged line surrounding the community. The health of a community at any time is on a continuum ranging from the optimal level of functioning to community dysfunction. An increase in self-care can lead to a higher state of functioning, and a decrease can lead to dysfunction. The optimal level of functioning is the "best functioning of the community, taking all things into account, it is the goal toward which communities strive."[5] Each community has an optimal level of functioning it strives to attain and to maintain. Dunn[6] explained that the achievement and maintenance of the optimal level of functioning requires

APPLICATION OF NURSING THEORIES

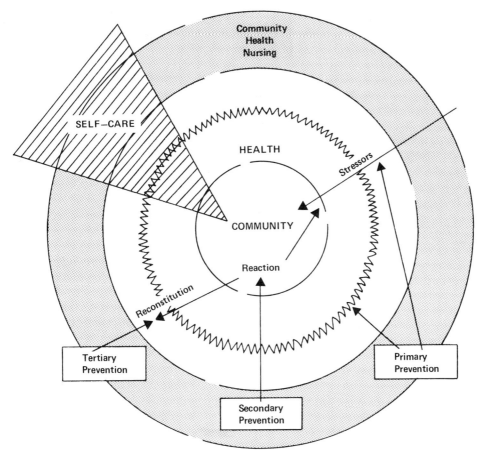

FIGURE 17-1. Diagram of the community health nursing model.

maintaining balance and purposeful direction. This closely parallels the notion that people must increase their self-care abilities to achieve a higher state of functioning.

Community health nursing is the practice of nursing with the community as the client; it is, according to Hamilton,[7] "the nursing of the community." The function of community health nursing is to promote the optimal level of community functioning through collaboration with members of the health care delivery service team and with members of the community. Consistent with the Neuman model, the model identifies the three intervention modes of primary, secondary, and tertiary prevention. In each of the modes community health nurses function by planning, advocating, coordinating, facilitating, educating, delivering, researching, managing, evaluating, and referring services.

The goal of primary prevention is to promote and to maintain the optimal level of functioning and to prevent decreased levels of functioning by focusing on the stressor to decrease it or to decrease the chance of the community's encountering the stressor or by focusing on the health state to increase the community's reacting ability. Secondary prevention is screening for early diagnosis of decreased functioning and prompt intervention to decrease the effects of a stressor. The focus of secondary prevention is the health state or the reaction process. The goal is to promote reconstitution (stability attainment) after a stressor is causing decreased health. Tertiary prevention occurs after treatment has resulted in reconstitution. Goals are to maintain stability and to promote the highest level of functioning possible by strengthening reaction to additional stressors and by preventing recurring reactions leading to regression on the continuum. Focus of tertiary prevention is on the reconstituted health state. The health state resulting from tertiary prevention can become the focus of primary prevention.[8]

The model presents the total view of the prevention modes in a circular fashion to illustrate that nursing interventions can begin at any of the intervention modes and can move in clockwise or counterclockwise directions as appropriate to promote health. The concept of self-care pervades each level of the nursing model. It acknowledges the population's right to be informed and to be knowledgeable about their health and encourages the community's independence and responsibility to provide its own self-care. As the client, the community becomes the decision maker and is provided the opportunity to make choices to act on its own behalf. Community health nurses can provide the support and expertise appropriate to these needs.[9]

Orem[10] suggests that the appropriate methods of helping communities are "guiding, providing psychological support, providing an environment for personal development, and teaching." These are consistent with our approach to community health nursing and serve as a sound philosophical base from which many of our decisions were based in meeting the needs of the gleaning community.

ASSESSMENT

Our interaction in the gleaning community was facilitated by the director of the area food bank, which served as the lead organization for several community projects, including gleaning in the tricounty metropolitan area. The director and several of the team leaders had identified potential health problems in the gleaning population related to the lack of first aid provisions at the pick sites and requested that a needs assessment be done on this community.

Using the community health nursing model, we could quickly get an idea of how this community perceived 1) stressors affecting its functioning, 2) its state of health and health care needs, and 3) its ability to meet its self-care needs. The community's perceptions about its health needs provide basic data about community interests and priorities. They often begin to identify areas of health care planning that community members will support.

A revised version of the Braden and Herban[11] model for community assessment was developed to approach this project and is illustrated in Figure 17-2.

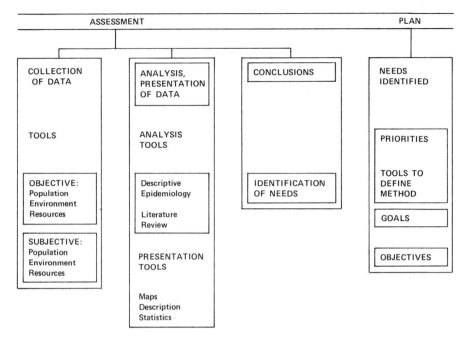

FIGURE 17-2. Diagram of model for community assessment. (Revised from Braden and Herban.[11]

The framework for this assessment includes the collection of data, analyses, presentation of data, and conclusions.

Braden and Herban[12] define assessment as "neither instant or static, but a continuous evolving process. It is the first step in problem identification and the initial step necessary for sound planning. Assessment is the planning undertaken to define or delineate need."

Assessment of the gleaning community was initiated using the key informant approach. After meeting the food bank director, we contacted key people within the organization who provided data we needed to begin the assessment. A meeting with the gleaning project directors was subsequently set up to discuss health needs as they perceived them. This approach enabled us to foster self-care in the community and to help the community population come together to identify its own needs and problem-solving abilities. As advocates for the community, we developed plans based on mutual acceptance to bring about changes in health care practices.

Gleaning file records of general information about the pickers was also made available to us. We reviewed the records and compiled the data about the population's age, families, size, sex, and any noted health problems.

Our model directed the development of a framework for assessment of the three community components identifying the following, which were considered in the assessment.

POPULATION AND ENVIRONMENT FACTORS
1. Population demographics
2. Population distribution
3. Health-illness status, patterns of disease, accidents, injuries
4. Psycho-social-cultural patterns
5. Physical environment characteristics
6. Biological-chemical environment
7. Social environment

RESOURCE FACTORS
1. Manpower
2. Transportation
3. Communication patterns
4. Financial resources
5. Political factors
6. Policies and procedures
7. Knowledge of resources
8. Health resources available
9. Accessibility of resources
10. Utilization of resources

Subjective and objective data were obtained to complete the assessment. The gathering of subjective data was achieved through interviews. Objective data were obtained by direct observation of the community and the review of records maintained by the group leaders. These tools provided a simple and workable guide which allowed us to focus our assessment process on obtaining the essential data about the community.

DATA COLLECTED

Environment

Not unlike other sites used for gleaning, this area was a wide-open field of strawberries and rhubarb, located in the southwestern part of the state. Surrounded by other open fields and accessible only by a dirt road, it extended to the highway. This area was subject to great plumes of dust created by the departure and arrival of cars loaded with pickers arriving in staggered shifts. There were very few trees in the immediate and adjacent areas, and only a few small sheds bordering on other fields. A crudely constructed outhouse stood in an open area at one end of the field, and no obvious facilities were available to accommodate handwashing. Weather conditions were somewhat favorable for picking—warm and sunny with a slight breeze blowing. Patches of the field were still muddy from recent rainfall in the area. The population of between 20 and 30 pickers varied in age and included children and senior citizens. They were predominantly female, adult, and no specific ethnic group was represented. The pickers were clad in various forms of attire, and very few wore hats for protection from the elements.

There was no discernible evidence of insects or rodents, although insect bites were a common complaint on previous picks. The knives distributed for cutting the rhubarb lay precariously about, presenting a hazard to all pickers, particularly children. No formal instructions were given to the pickers regarding safety in the field.

Pickers assumed a variety of positions for gleaning, lifting, and transporting the produce, with little regard to proper body mechanics. No water or food was available at the site, and pickers were expected to provide for their own nutritional needs.

Population

In the areas we assessed, the gleaning population grew from 1310 in 1980 to more than 4000 in 1981. Each group had one project director, 20 to 30 field bosses or team leaders, and a board of directors made up of volunteers who are legally responsible for the program.

A sample population of 599 being served by this program was taken from the records on file. A summary of the findings indicated they were predominantly female, between the ages of 18 and 64. Health problems were difficult to identify owing to poor response from the participants.

The records were devoid of pertinent information to assess the health problems of this population with any accuracy. There were no methods being used to acquire such data as education level, ethnic group, morbidity, mortality, or accidents in the field.

Both formal and informal patterns of communication were used effectively by the gleaners. The informal pattern included a telephone tree. The project director was notified of the pick by the farmer, and information was forwarded to the team leaders by phone. The message was relayed to the rest of the community by each one calling another, and arrangements for babysitting and transportation were made informally at this time. Formal channels of communication were operating through traditional media, such as television, radio, telephone, and interagency bulletins.

Resources

Financial resources included a recently acquired small United Way grant. These monies were placed under the control of the community council of the food bank to cover the cost of a coordinator's salary, mailing, travel expenses, and supplies. Finances were indirectly obtained through the use of volunteers and trade for services with community merchants. Trade for service is an exchange of services between merchants and volunteer gleaners whereby no direct funds are exchanged. Efforts to raise significant amounts of money through bake sales, yard sales, and so forth were not successful.

Interfaces with political systems were evident by the procurement of United Way funds and the federal tax write-off for farmers participating in the program. Local television, radio, and newspapers provided avenues to increase public awareness of the program and its purpose.

Health resources, facilities, and personnel available were found to be inadequate for this population. Gleaners in the field had to travel long distances to obtain health care. There were no first aid kits at the sites in case of accidents or emergencies, and there were no trained personnel to provide care. There were no existing protocols established for emergency care to the sick or injured. The accessibility of health care services was limited because of lack of knowledge of available community resources, low income, and inability to use existing health care systems.

Conclusion

Analysis of the data indicated a high potential for health-related problems for the population in this environment. The impetus of gleaners to become part of the rural community was necessitated by insufficient incomes to buy the food they needed. With average yearly incomes below the poverty level, these low-income groups lacked the buying power to provide adequate diets for their existence. As Leahy, Cobb, and Jones[13] point out, poverty is often perceived as a health hazard because of inadequate nutrition and insufficient medical care, which, in turn, make the poor more vulnerable to poor health and the inabilities to cope with it.

Emergency health care for this community was lacking, and a special emphasis for providing this service was needed. During our meetings with the gleaners, the need expressed time and time again was for members to become trained to administer first aid to gleaners in the field in emergency situations.

The organization's records were deficient of pertinent information to validate the health problems inherent to this group. There was a pressing need to provide a mechanism to record the incidence of problems and to provide the support for what needed to be done.

Clearly, this community lacked the ability to obtain the health services it needed. There was limited use of community resources and limited knowledge of how to arrange for the first aid training they needed. The community's preoccupation with gleaning preempted the need for health care, and the lack of qualified people to administer first aid was not recognized until an emergency situation occurred on one of the picks.

By its own design, areas for gleaning are not easily accessible to health care facilities. They are in rural areas accessible only by access roads from the freeway and are several miles from most health care facilities. This is a major consideration when injuries or illnesses require immediate attention. The nature of tho environment lends itself to health hazards and accidents and the need for emergency service.

Analysis of the subjective and objective data led to the identification of health needs for the gleaning community. Our model identifies health needs as the stressors having impact on the health of the community. These needs were considered in terms of priority, using the tool we developed from the Risk Factor Analysis Model presented by Decker[14] and our conceptual model for nursing. The tool is presented in Table 17-1. Each identified need was scored as high, medium, or low in six categories. The categories are the community's perception of the priority level of the need, the degree of community system reaction caused by the need, the feasibility of modifying the need, the probability of decreasing the need by modifying contributing factors, the number of people affected by the need, and the overall priority level of the need.

By using this tool, we labeled five high-priority needs, three medium-priority needs, and three low-priority needs.

To present our recommendations we met with the gleaners and jointly discussed and agreed upon the following list of needs.

HIGH PRIORITY
1. Lack of first aid kits at pick sites
2. Lack of first aid training/knowledge
3. Lack of guidelines for actions for emergencies, injuries, illnesses
   a. Potential for acute trauma; for example, cardiac arrest, wounds, fractures, accidents, heat exhaustion, respiratory distress, insect bites
   b. Incidence of hypertension, diabetes, heart disease, respiratory disease, musculoskeletal problems in the population
4. Environmental hazards related to health
   a. Transportation-related (for example, road accidents, parking lot hazards), equipment, inappropriate clothing, overexposure to elements, improper body mechanics, lack of preventative methods such as insect repellents, sunscreens
5. Lack of health information owing to inadequate registration forms for participants
MEDIUM PRIORITY
1. Lack of drinking water at pick site
2. Lack of sanitation facilities (handwashing facilities) at pick site
3. Lack of appropriate emergency food/nutrition supply at pick site
LOW PRIORITY
1. Underutilization of resources
   a. Lack of knowledge and understanding of internal and external resources
   b. Barriers to utilization
   c. Lack of advocate for obtaining health resources
2. Lack of financial resources

TABLE 17-1. Priority Tool

NEED	COMMUNITY PERCEPTION OF PRIORITY LEVEL	DEGREE OF REACTION	FEASIBILITY OF MODIFYING NEED	PROBABILITY OF DECREASING NEED BY MODIFYING FACTORS	NUMBER OF PEOPLE AFFECTED	OVERALL PRIORITY LEVEL
1. Lack of first aid kits	High	High	High	High	High	High
2. Lack of training and knowledge	High	High	High	High	High	High
3. Lack of guidelines	High	High	High	High	High	High
4. Environmental hazards—actual and potential	Medium	High	High	High	High	High
5. Lack of drinking water	Low	Medium	High	Medium	High	Medium
6. Lack of sanitation facilities	Low	Low	High	Medium	High	Medium
7. Lack of emergency food supply	Low	High	High	Medium	Medium	Medium
8. Incomplete forms	Medium	Medium	High	High	Low	Medium
9. Underutilization of resources	Low	Low	Medium	High	High	High
10. Lack of group cohesiveness	Medium	Medium	Low	Low	Medium	Low
					Low	Low

INTERVENTIONS

With the needs identified, the development of our plan to meet these needs began. With the assistance of the coordinator of the American Red Cross first aid class, we developed a list of necessary supplies for the gleaners' first aid kits. We investigated resources for low-cost supplies and obtained donated bandages from the Red Cross. A "quick check list" for gleaners was designed to be a quick reference card which would guide gleaners to provide for their own safety and self-care during picks. We developed a field boss instruction sheet related to health and safety at the pick site. The gleaning registration form was revised to include more categories for obtaining information on the health status, ethnic group, and yearly income of program participants. We used Red Cross reference information to compile the booklet of guidelines for action in first aid emergencies.

We made repeated contacts with the American Red Cross to facilitate the enrollment of the gleaners in first aid and cardiopulmonary resuscitation (CPR) courses. Our meeting with the director of the safety division resulted in the Red Cross offering first aid courses to gleaners at a reduced rate.

We obtained and delivered to the community representatives information about first aid class times and registration procedures. We also arranged and attended a meeting during which the gleaning program coordinator, as the community liaison, and the Red Cross course coordinator worked out a planned method for ongoing use of Red Cross services by the gleaning community. Through our interventions the community will be able to arrange independently to have the field bosses trained in first aid and in CPR.

As the final activity of implementation, we explored with the community the idea of seeking a community health nurse as an advisory board member. A community health nurse could serve as a consultant and advocate for the community's future efforts to assess and to meet health needs. The gleaners responded positively to this discussion and indicated that they could arrange for ongoing interaction with a nurse.

Twelve gleaners attended the first class in first aid offered to the gleaners. The cooperative effort to promote health and safety was evident by the enthusiastic response of the Red Cross staff and gleaning community.

The Red Cross has strongly encouraged the gleaning population to enroll in the free CPR classes it is offering as part of a major CPR training program. The gleaning program coordinator acted as the liaison between the Red Cross and the gleaners to promote enrollment in these and future CPR and first aid courses.

In retrospect, there were many steps in this process that proved effective. One is the close collaboration with the gleaners during the process. We frequently met to validate information, to receive input, to make decisions, and to define roles and expectations. Our systematic approach to this project was another positive aspect. It allowed us to be organized and efficient in our planning and delineated the steps for clear direction. Our model tells us that the community health nurse works at three levels of prevention. Most of our interventions were at the primary and secondary level. It is significant to note that the three levels of prevention are cyclic and used when appropriate.

Getting into the system was an effective measure and could be attributed to our ability to relate to the gleaners at their level and to recognize the needs as they perceived them. Time did not allow us to interview other gleaners who might have provided input from a different perspective and might have helped us establish a broad assessment base of the target population.

The major limitations to this project were the time allowed to accomplish the task and the lack of data available in the program's records. Files were devoid of data in many significant areas. We were confined to using the key informant approach to assessment because of the reluctance of the population to respond to a survey questionnaire. This limited our primary source of data. These limitations could be overcome through the gleaning community's ongoing interaction with a community health nurse consultant.

The experience of using our model was new and exciting. It served as a guide to our practice by providing a systematic method for assessing a community and further defined the role of the community health nurse. It is our concerted belief, however, that further testing and development of the model is needed.

REFERENCES

1. MEAD, S: Gleaning in Oregon: The experiment grows. Community Food Report, April 1, 1982, pp 3–4.

2. OREM, DE: Nursing: Concepts of Practice, ed 2. McGraw-Hill, New York, 1980, p 35.

3. WILLIAMS, CA: Community health nursing—what is it? Nurs Outlook 25(4):250, 1977.

4. CLEMEN, SA, EIGSTI, DG, McGUIRE, SL: Comprehensive Family and Community Health Nursing. McGraw-Hill, New York, 1981.

5. ARCHER, SE AND FLESHMAN, RP: Community Health Nursing Patterns and Practice, ed 2. Duxbury Press, North Scituate, MA, 1979, p 34.

6. DUNN, H: High-Level Wellness. RW Beatle, Arlington, VA, 1961.

7. HAMILTON, P: Community nursing diagnosis. ANS, April 1983, p 30.

8. NEUMAN, B: The Neuman Systems Model—Application to Nursing Education and Practice. Appleton-Century-Crofts, Norwalk, CT, 1982.

9. SULLIVAN, TJ: Self-care model for nursing. New Directions for Nursing in the 80's. American Nurses Association, Kansas City, MO, 1980.

10. OREM, op cit, p 61.

11. BRADEN, CJ AND HERBAN, NL: *Community Health: A Systems Approach.* Appleton-Century-Crofts, New York, 1976.

12. Ibid, p 63.

13. LEAHY, K, COBB, M, JONES, M: *Community Health Nursing*, ed 2. McGraw-Hill, New York, 1966.

14. DECKER, S: *Risk factor analysis model.* Unpublished class notes, N504, University of Portland Graduate Nursing School, Summer 1982.

CHAPTER 18

COMMUNITY ASSESSMENT USING ROY'S MODEL

SHERRY BENNETT HOWARD, R.N., M.S.

A nurse who works in a hospital may use concepts of community assessment to determine the health care needs of the community serviced by that hospital. The hospital may be viewed as a health service provider in relation to the community client just as the community health nurse is a health service provider.

It is of paramount importance to have a clear and appropriate concept of a community as a client. Karp[1] views the community client as a population aggregate with three elements: 1) a geographical area; 2) members bound together by a common attribute, whether it be values or goals; and 3) members engaged in sustained social interaction.

This broad definition easily allows a hospital to be denoted as a community and to exist within a community. Planning for the future has become an important focus of hospitals so that they can provide services for the community and respond to their needs more efficiently and cost effectively. In order for a hospital administration to make sound decisions to provide direction for the years ahead, it must look at the community in which the hospital is located. A needs assessment provides the information necessary to look at who the hospital serves, who it should serve, and which services to implement. A nurse in a hospital using the community health nursing's concept of community as a client is qualified to originate and to implement a needs assessment that leads to a description, analysis, and recommendations for future services to the community the hospital serves based on health care trends.

This chapter describes how a nurse, as a member of a hospital's management team, used a conceptual framework for community assessment. A conceptual framework guides the process by providing a structure in which concepts, facts, theories, and propositions are united. In order to apply a framework, it is first necessary to capture a view of the "working insides" of the conceptual framework. Three key areas provide this guidance for the practice of community health nursing: They are management principles, the health planning process, and a nursing model.

ROY'S ADAPTATION MODEL OF NURSING

Roy's Adaptation Model of nursing provides guidance to delivery of service to the community. The following discussion will include selected aspects of Roy's model and additional theories for community application. The community is seen as the adaptive system. Roy's model represents a system's model and identifies the recipient of nursing care as a biopsychosocial adaptive system.[2] In simplest terms, that involves input, processes, feedback, and output.[3] A system is open, with permeable boundaries that exchange with subsystems and suprasystems functioning by the interdependence of its parts.[4] It is important to use "systems" terminology because many disciplines use a systems theory orientation in looking at communities. This will foster communication, increase nursing's credibility, and overall enhance the ability to work together.

Roy and Roberts[5] describe adaptation as a positive response to a continually changing internal and external environment that ultimately will promote self-mastery. This changing environment is the input for the community as an open system and has been termed stimuli.

The focal stimulus is the one to which the community must make a response which, it is hoped, will be adaptive in nature. It is the stimulus most immediately confronting the community. Roy discusses mediating factors as those which contribute to the effect of the focal stimulus. These mediating factors are contextual stimuli, which are all other stimuli present, and residual stimuli (that is, beliefs, experiences), which are those stimuli affecting the situation but not easily validated or measured.[6]

Adaptive responses are a function of the confronting stimuli and the adaptation level. The pooled effect of the three classes of stimuli determine the adaptation level. It is a constantly changing point that represents the standard of the range of stimuli that the community will tolerate with ordinary adaptive responses. Stimuli might be economical, sociological, ecological, or political in nature. A health problem could also be a stimulus confronting the community.

The adaptive system uses coping mechanisms to maintain stability by processing information. The human system has two major internal processor mechanisms: the regulator and the cognator. The regulator works through the autonomic nervous system, which readies the person for coping via a reflex action of flight or fight. The cognator assists the person consciously by means of thought and decision and unconsciously through the defense mechanisms by identifying, storing, and relating stimuli so that symbolic responses can be made.[7]

These coping mechanisms act in relation to the following four modes: 1) physiological needs, which involve the body's basic needs; 2) self-concept, which is the composite of beliefs and feelings one holds about oneself at a given time; 3) role function, which is the performance of duties based on a given position in society; and 4) interdependence, which means a balance between dependence and independence (that is, a need for nurturing but also self-sufficiency).[8]

The concept of coping has been expanded to include culture as the mechanism used by the community to cope. Culture is the means by which human systems interpret their experiences and guide their actions. It refers to shared ideas, values, and behaviors in a dynamic state which provide a sense of security; without having to think, one knows how to act. The culture is seen as the "brain" of the community, because it stores learned information, attitudes, and beliefs. It processes data for decision making.[9-13] Roy and Roberts[14] offer support to an expansion of the model in their latest text by stating that the notion of adaptation is applicable to the community but needs further theorizing about inputs, coping mechanisms, and outputs.

This necessity for expansion extends to the identification of the modes of adaptation which provide the manifestation of the coping mechanism's activity. In this case, the coping mechanism is the concept of culture, and it acts in relation to the modes of adaptation. Roy[15] suggested that the adaptive modes for a community client might be the five functions of a community as denoted by Warren. These functions are production-distribution-consumption, socialization, social control, social participation, and mutual support.[16]

Production-distribution-consumption provides work, goods, and services as accessible commodities. Exchange of goods and services takes place not only within communities but among them. For example, patient care is the service offered by a hospital community. Secondly, socialization is the process of learning through which individuals acquire values, knowledge, and behaviors appropriate to social role functioning. The community is not the only factor in the socialization process but does have a continuing role throughout time to maintain social roles which pattern social behavior. Education is a good example of an effector of socialization. The third function, social control, is the process through which influences toward conformity of norms are visualized. This controlling process is usually internalized as one's "conscience" if the individual sees it as important. All levels of government perform this function. Fourthly, social participation is simply the relating of people to one another (that is, friendships, membership in organizations). Finally, mutual support is the type of assistance that is preferred in those instances of needs not being met in the usual pattern of organized social behavior (for example, illness or economic distress).

These adaptive modes are interrelated, one affecting the other. The effective or ineffective functioning of the community's culture in response to a stimulus is manifested in these five functions. It is hoped that this response is adaptive in that needs are met or goals are attained. At this point there may be unexpected outcomes, such as new problems being identified or problems not previously identified being solved through the problem/service.

Whatever the response, it acts as feedback into the system as growth for coping with future internal or external environmental stimuli.[17] One can see adaptation as an ongoing process within the scope of the feedback mechanism, as well as an end-state solution to a problem. This entire process puts the community somewhere on the health-illness continuum.

These concepts are denoted in Figure 18-1, a diagram of this conceptual framework. The last critical component that has not been discussed yet, as depicted in the diagram, is the role of the community health nurse.

Nursing's goal is to promote community adaptation in regard to the adaptive modes. The nurse intervenes by working *with* the community to bring the stimuli into the community's adaptation zone so that positive coping can occur. The adaptation level sets up this zone to indicate the extent of stimuli that will elicit a positive response. Stimuli that fall outside this zone cause a negative response. An adaptive response maintains integrity, and an ineffective response does not lead to goal attainment or it disrupts integrity.[18] This means that the nurse may have to increase, decrease, or modify the stimuli. By solving or pre-

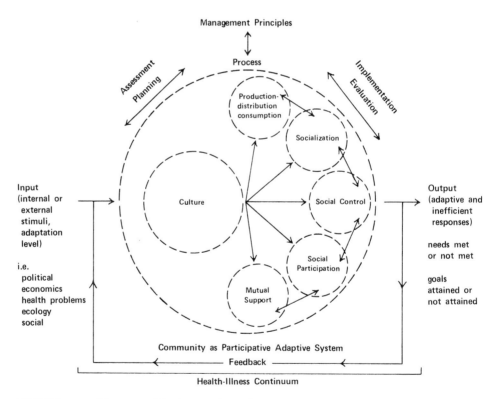

FIGURE 18-1. Diagram of the integration of Nursing, Community, and Adaptation concepts. (Adapted from Roy, Sister Callista: *Adaptation Model.* Supplementary Material for Nurse Theorist General Session, Second Annual Nurse Educator Conference, New York, December, 1978.)

venting problems, the community is free to respond to the other stimuli. When energy is freed from inadequate coping attempts, it will contribute to overall higher-level wellness. An example of prevention of health problems is community immunization programs. Because the community does not have to control epidemics, it can devote its energy toward solving or preventing other problems.

Roy and Roberts[19] state that when unusual stresses or weakened coping mechanisms make the community's usual attempts to cope ineffective, then a nurse is needed. That is true, but the role of the nurse should also be to prevent the stimuli from falling outside the adaptation zone initially. Roy does not address the preventative focus in depth. This is an important consideration when applying this model to community assessment, because the community health nurse views prevention of health problems as a major priority.

Roy and Roberts[20] discuss White's contention that adaptive responses are more likely if the community can keep securing adequate information about the environment, maintain satisfactory internal conditions for processing information and taking action, and maintain autonomy to function in a flexible manner. The nurse participates with the community to promote adaptive responses through the health planning process, which is comparable with the nursing process.

HEALTH PLANNING PROCESS	NURSING PROCESS
Data gathering, analysis, goal setting	Assessment
Planning	Planning
Strategies for achieving goals	Implementation
Evaluation	Evaluation

The concepts are interchangeable, although the terms are different. The health planning process is aimed at population aggregates and may take longer to implement and to see the end result.

The process begins with an assessment of data, leads to an analysis, and results in goal setting. Through this the planner can clearly identify problems or potential problems. The type and amount of data to be collected will depend on differing situations, but it must be recognized that every bit of knowledge will help. Time constraints and data overload cannot be ignored, though.

A community assessment can be used to determine the community's strengths, weaknesses, placement on the health-illness continuum, interpretation of incoming stimuli, and the adaptive modes. One can find numerous assessment tools for the nurse to use in the nursing literature or the nurse may develop his or her own. The assessment tool at the end of this chapter depicts an approach for organizing data and correlates with the expansion of Roy's model previously presented. This tool is unique in that it not only provides a form for organizing universal data that should be collected when assessing a community but has a focus for the nurse who uses Roy's Adaptation Model of nursing. The methods for collecting these data are varied, such as census data, key informants, surveys, and vital statistics. Reference texts assist the nurse to choose the most appropriate tools depending on individual situations.

COMMUNITY NEEDS ASSESSMENT

The conceptual framework presented here is applied to a long-range planning process undertaken at a hospital in the Northwest. For the sake of simplicity, this hospital will be referred to as NW Hospital.

The community health nurse began the planning process with a needs assessment. The data collected and presented here are limited because of time constraints, but they provide an overview for showing this conceptual framework's applicability.

NW Hospital is a 195-bed nonprofit, general acute-care hospital with medical, surgical, and psychiatric facilities. The Neuropsychiatric Center is one of the largest and most modern psychiatric units in the Northwest, having 52 beds. The oncology unit provides 12 beds, and the rehabilitation unit consists of six beds. The hospital is located on the east side of the city between a coliseum and a major shopping center and is readily accessible from all sections of the city by freeway and main streets. In 1981, a House Calls Program was established by the hospital to provide physician services to patients in their homes. The concept is unique to the city and innovative in the sense that a hospital is the sponsor. A Sports Medicine Center is a new aspect of the hospital.

NW Hospital has evolved since 1893. In 1920, it was the first veteran's hospital in the city. After 13 years as a veteran's hospital, the name was changed to NW Hospital. In 1940, a psychiatric center was established to serve a community need. In addition, when polio became an epidemic in the 1950s, NW Hospital became the center for patients using "iron lungs." NW Hospital has kept and is continuing to keep pace with medical advances to provide quality patient care services.

NW Hospital is located in a high-density, complex, mature port city whose shipping activities have impact on the state's economy. An intense effort has been undertaken by city leaders to revitalize the business core after a tremendous population migration to surrounding suburban areas. The city has experienced a shortage of housing in the downtown area and in the urban neighborhoods owing to redevelopment efforts. The city council established a housing policy to replace lost housing, to rehabilitate existing housing, and to create new single-family and multifamily housing.

The total number of jobs in the city is increasing, and greater percentages are being taken by suburban residents. Ready access to public transportation and the ability of freeways and major arterials to accommodate an increase in automobiles are planned. A rapid transit system and another bridge will lessen downtown freeway congestion and provide easier access to the city.

It is estimated that the city's population has decreased by 10,000 people in the past 10 years, and a continued slow decrease is anticipated. The population groups within the city are diverse, and most of the area's ethnic minorities and low-income, elderly, and single young adults are concentrated there.

Review of census data provides the following description of the characteristics of the city's population: 77.9 percent of the city's population have at least a high school diploma, and college degrees are held by 22 percent of the population over 25 years of age, with 20 percent holding higher degrees.

Considering racial distributions, the area is 90 percent Caucasian, 5 percent black, 3 percent Asians and Pacific Islanders, and 2 percent other races. There are 2.55 persons per household, and the average number of people in the family is 3.10. There are more female heads of households than male.

The work force in 1979 was employed mainly by manufacturing, secondly by services, and thirdly by retail trade. Median family income for Caucasians was $22,357, for blacks $14,490, and for Asians and Pacific Islanders $20,695. Out of 949,430 people over the age of 16, 626,648 are deemed to be in the civilian work force. Of these, 589,090 are employed, and 37,558 are unemployed, accounting for an average of 6 percent unemployment.

In 1980, the elderly population (age 65 and over) comprised approximately 13 percent of the population. Estimates put this percentage at 18.3 percent by 1990. This figure will increase significantly over the next 30 to 50 years as the 18 to 64 age group ages (currently accounting for 63 percent of the planning area population).

The core of the city has the oldest and largest hospitals, the highest concentration of medical manpower, and the most specialized services. The city's hospitals tend to be large, vertical, and few—perhaps because the city is so concentrated in a tight geographical area, with land at a premium.

An assessment of existing resources indicates that there are five large hospitals in this area, each with a total capacity of over 450 beds. Tertiary services range from neurosurgery, open-heart surgery, renal dialysis, and radiation oncology. These hospitals are also considered the teaching and research centers for the area, ranging from ownership arrangements of a state university system to the federal government.

In addition, there are five other hospitals in the city ranging from 50 to 250 beds. One of these hospitals serves a preenrolled population. Although this hospital serves a larger portion of the population from the area, each of the other four hospitals serves less than 5 percent of the population.

Three additional hospitals outside the immediate city area each serve more than 5 percent of the population. What can be said with some certainty is that no new urban hospitals are needed and that not all existing hospitals should be replaced as they become outmoded.

The demographic data are a vital base for the planning process. In order to plan effectively, it is important to know historical and current information about the internal and external environments of the hospital. A Northwest Council of Hospitals (NCH) responded to a lack of planning by hospitals by producing a Hospital Development Guide to enhance understanding of hospital systems and to aid the process of planning for the community's health needs.

Planning areas are identified to assist in planning services but are not a set of fixed boundaries defining a hospital's responsibilities and services for a specified population area. Patients use services outside the boundaries of planning areas, reflecting free choice, service availability, and doctors' preference. The hospital's market share is determined by measuring the percentages of discharges from each hospital as compared with that planning area's total number of discharges and the percentages of each hospital's discharges from each planning area. NW Hospital's market share of the planning area shows that 56.2 percent of the patients come from the immediate geographic area.

A service area analysis, or an analysis of where patients come from for existing services, is vital to examine. Northwest Hospital has the highest concentration of discharges (47.2 percent) from 11 zip codes in the immediate area. A secondary service area is identified by additional zip codes, representing 33.3 percent of discharges. The zip code in which NW Hospital is located accounts for 4.4 percent of discharges.

When Roy's model is applied in analyzing the implications of the assessment data for NW Hospital, the following conclusions may be drawn. The most significant stimulus confronting NW Hospital at this time is the economic scene. The solvency of this institution is dependent upon usage by clients. The impetus for the patient origin study that is analyzed here is the hospital's response to a changing environment. It is important to know where clients are coming from so that planning can take place for future service development, maintenance, or depletion.

Contextual and residual stimuli that affect the hospital at any one time are numerous and varied. They may become focal stimuli, depending on the situation and the strengths and weaknesses of the internal environment. A few of the stimuli are the threat of increased governmental regulation, increased usage of day surgery in lieu of inpatient services, nursing staff's demand for better wages and respect from other disciplines, decreased ability of clients to pay hospital bills, and the taking over of administrative functioning by an outside management firm.

NW Hospital's usual method of coping with problems or planning to prevent problems, and the strength of the stimulus confronting the hospital, will dictate whether the culture of the community will produce adaptive responses. For the continued existence of the hospital, it will be vital that the majority of responses be speedily adaptive. Within this dramatically changing time hospitals are closing.

The hospital community is functioning in the five adaptive modes. At this time, the culture is probably using coping strategies to deal with economic instability in the way that it has in the past. Having a short time to study NW Hospital, one could view only a limited part of the hospital's learned behavior and way of decision making. It is probable that this hospital has always had to respond to economic stimuli (for example the expansion and modernization of other hospitals in the city to capture a greater share of the market). As these responses were successful or unsuccessful, they fed back into the system for a different level functioning.

Some of the behaviors seen in the adaptive modes are described below.

1. *Production-distribution-consumption.* The service of providing patient care is marketed through activities such as the public relations depart-

ment, new program development, physicians' clients, and client-to-client word of mouth.

2. *Socialization.* In these times of economic need, the hospital is learning new behaviors to survive (for example, tighter budget control by guiding/educating the department heads about cost-effectiveness or zero-based budgeting).

3. *Social control.* In this mode, it is vital to mention the effect of the supra-system (government) on hospitals. The issue of the day is health care cost inflation, and hospitals and physicians cannot ignore the pressure of conforming to cost control any longer.

4. *Social participation.* Employees participate in meetings outside and inside the hospital to foster relationships to deal with the demands being put upon them.

5. *Mutual support.* The hospital was just taken over by an outside management firm, perhaps to help it deal with needs not being met in usual ways. It also has a long-range planner to assist with meeting needs.

CONCLUSIONS AND RECOMMENDATIONS

From analyzing the data collected in the needs assessment, one can determine that NW Hospital is still surviving or responding in an adaptive fashion at this time. The demographic data, health care trends, market and service area analysis, and "tight" economic times lead to recommendations that will expand existing services and meet needs not already being met by other hospitals and that will be cost effective. To prevent inefficient coping responses in the future by NW Hospital, the following initial recommendations were generated from the assessment. These would require further investigation to determine their appropriateness and priority.

1. Establish a home health outreach program.
   Rationale: The aged population is increasing. The trend will be away from hospital care to home care. NW Hospital already has a psychiatric clientele that requires follow up at home. With decreasing government funding to mental health centers, the hospital could expand its services to meet this community need. The House Calls Program would be another source for clients for home health, because many of the clients are elderly without help at home.

2. Establish exercise programs for the public through the sports medicine program.
   Rationale: Expanding the sports medicine program would not be increasing costs to the hospital and yet could meet a community need that other hospitals are not already meeting. People are becoming wellness oriented through education and peer pressure. Health awareness is be-

ing encouraged for patients by their physicians; therefore, physician referrals can become a source of clients. Health clubs are springing up throughout the city but are usually staffed by inadequately educated personnel. The staff at the hospital are candidates who could insure safe exercise programs. Other programs might be weight control and stress reduction.

3. Establish outreach programs in the areas of stress management, financial management, and occupational therapy through the neuropsychiatric center.
   Rationale: The Neuropsychiatric Center already conducts similar programs within the hospital.

4. Expand the present day-care program for hospital personnel to an outreach program into the community to serve preschool children of all working parents.
   Rationale: The work force of women is increasing, and NW Hospital already has trained personnel to do this job. All the aforementioned recommendations will increase the visibility of the hospital, thus it should have a "ripple effect."

5. Conduct a needs assessment and resource utilization of the immediate zip code area in which NW Hospital is located.
   Rationale: Ascertain why the hospital is not receiving more patients from this area. From this data, a plan for future services responsive to the needs of this area could be developed.

In addition to the recommendations derived from the assessment, the long-range planner for the hospital was already investigating the possibility for developing programs in industrial medicine and alcohol rehabilitation to meet the needs of the immediate area, inasmuch as it is a highly industrialized section of the city.

After analysis of collected data identification of problems or potential problems and study of initial recommendation, the next step is planning. This part of the process provides action toward an outcome through priority determination, goal setting, and objective definition. Alternative solutions for meeting goals and objectives are generated, and appropriate actions are determined. Planning, it is hoped, is most often done to anticipate problems rather than to solve existing problems. In planning for intervention, one should consider the community, resources, and constraints. Spiegel and Hyman[21] discuss tools useful in priority setting. One such tool is the Simplex method, in which scored structured questions are used to analyze each problem or solution and top priority is given to the ones with the highest numbers.

The briefness of the discussion here on planning in no way denotes its importance. Its importance cannot be stressed enough because it leads us into the implementation phase, which is the action aspect. One can see how in the assessment, planning, and implementation phases, the principles of management are interrelated. The skills used during the implementation phase are directing, coordinating, staffing, and organizing resources. Implementation is a process of change, so abilities as a change agent, good communicator, negotiator, teacher, consultant, and so forth become the nurses' power armamentarium.

The final phase is evaluation, an integral part of the decision-making process. Braden and Herban[22] describe evaluation as a process of determining the amount of success in achieving a predetermined objective, including the steps of formulation, identifying criteria for measurement, determining and explaining the degree of success, and formulating recommendations for future activities. From this definition, it can be seen that this process is cyclic in nature.

In asking what impact the implementation of a plan has had, one may use different vehicles, again depending on the situation. Spiegel and Hyman[23] discuss the National Health Planning Act of 1974. This act suggested the following six categories to measure impact:

1. Acceptability: Is the community satisfied and complying?
2. Accessibility: Are there any barriers, such as transportation or language?
3. Availability of personnel and services
4. Continuity of care through referral systems
5. Cost
6. Qualities of facilities, of personnel, of process, and of outcome.

Braden and Herban[24] suggest that after evaluation occurs, reassessment and reprogramming to meet current and projected needs must be used to adapt continually. The four stages of health planning are interwoven strands.

The hospital as a client of a community health nurse is exciting and challenging when one looks at the questions and ideas that can be generated from health care trends. Should the hospital open an extended-care facility to meet the need of decreased nursing-home beds? Should the hospital market itself for prepaid hospital plans? Can a hospice program be coordinated through the hospital inpatient department?

These and many more questions can be answered for hospital administration through the long-range planning process which incorporates the use of a needs assessment. Community health nurses can conduct a needs assessment as a basis for the planning process. To aid in this task, the nurse can use a nursing model like the one presented here to promote the hospital's adaptability in these rapidly changing times. Using a nursing model to guide one's practice will enhance the development of the model.

ASSESSMENT TOOL FOR ADAPTATION FRAMEWORK

AGENCY PERFORMING ASSESSMENT

Name _____ Size _____

Address and type _____

Organizational structure _____

Historical background _____

Manpower _____
Money sources _____

Goals _____
How evaluation of service accomplished _____

COMMUNITY
Location and Population
    Country _____
    State _____
    County _____
    City _____
Sexes _____   Birth Rate _____
Marital Status _____   Race _____
Mortality Rate _____   Income _____
Migration Patterns _____
Education Level _____   Immunization Level _____
Social/ethnic background _____
Occupation _____
Ages _____
Transportation _____
Utilities _____
Communication systems _____

Recreational activities _____
Motels/hotels _____
Existing facilities (including health care) _____
Geophysical characteristics _____
Housing _____
Number of people per household _____   Number of people per family _____
Leading causes of death _____   Chronic diseases _____
Communicable diseases _____   _____
_____   _____

Social Climate _____   Perception of time _____
Social Problems _____
Focal Stimuli _____
Contextual Stimuli _____
Residual Stimuli _____
Culture _____
Religious beliefs _____
Marketing strategies _____

Governmental influence _____

Political affiliations _____

Psychological stability _____ Physiological stability _____

Sociological stability _____

Production-distribution-consumption _____

Socialization _____

Social control _____

Social participation _____

Mutual support _____

Other _____

REFERENCES

1. KARP, DA: *Being Urban: Social, Psychological View of City Life.* DC Heath, Lexington, MA, 1977.

2. RIEHL, JP AND ROY, C: *Conceptual Models for Nursing Practice,* ed 2. Appleton-Century-Crofts, New York, 1980.

3. BRADEN, CJ AND HERBAN, NL: *Community Health: A Systems Approach.* Appleton-Century-Crofts, New York, 1976.

4. HALL, JE AND WEAVER, BR: *Distributive Nursing Practice: A Systems Approach to Community Health.* JB Lippincott, Philadelphia, 1977.

5. ROY, SC AND ROBERTS, SL: *Theory Construction in Nursing: An Adaptation Model.* Prentice-Hall, Englewood Cliffs, NJ, 1981.

6. ROY, SC: *Adaptation: A basis for nursing practice.* Nurs Outlook 19:254, 1971.

7. ROY, SC: *Adaptation: A conceptual framework for nursing.* Nurs Outlook 18:42, 1970.

8. Ibid.

9. BRADEN AND HERBAN, op cit.

10. HALL AND WEAVER, op cit.

11. HELVIE, C: *Community Health Nursing Theory and Process.* Harper & Row, Philadelphia, 1981.

12. LEAHY, K, COBB, M, JONES, M: *Community Health Nursing,* ed 3. McGraw-Hill, New York, 1977.

13. SPRADLEY, BW: *Community Health Nursing Concepts and Practice.* Little, Brown & Co, Boston, 1981.

14. ROY AND ROBERTS, op cit.

15. ROY, SC: Personal communication, July 1982.

16. WARREN, R: *The Community in America.* Rand McNally, Chicago, 1963.

17. Roy, SC: *Adaptation: A conceptual framework for nursing,* op cit.

18. Roy and Roberts, op cit.

19. Roy and Roberts, op cit.

20. Roy and Roberts, op cit.

21. Spiegel, A and Hyman, H: *Basic Health Planning Methods.* Aspen, Germantown, MD, 1978.

22. Braden and Herban, op cit.

23. Spiegel and Hyman, op cit.

24. Braden and Herban, op cit.

CHAPTER 19

MARTHA ROGERS'S MODEL: AN INTERPRETATION AND APPLICATION

CAROL ALLEN, R.N., M.S.

A variety of conceptual approaches can be applied to the assessment of a community. The approach chosen determines the type of data collected and ultimately the nursing diagnoses, outcome criteria, and interventions which are generated.[1] A conceptual framework developed from a nursing perspective is most likely to address nursing's concerns. Martha Rogers, a nurse who has an extensive educational and experiential background in community health, has developed a conceptual framework that reflects nursing's central concerns—person, environment, nursing, and health—in a uniquely holistic, optimistic, and futuristic way.[2]

Rogers's model represents an application of a new paradigm which emerged from quantum mechanics in physics and has subsequently been used to describe the natural and human world. The cornerstone of this view is that humans and their environments are irreducible whole energy fields in continuous mutual, simultaneous interaction with an open universe unbounded by space or time.[3]

This chapter will describe the four essential building blocks of Rogers's theory: energy fields, four-dimensionality, pattern and organization, and the life process. The three principles of homeodynamics—resonancy, integrality, and helicy—which emerge from this view and provide direction to the nurse in the application of the nursing process will also be described. Finally, the model will be applied to the assessment of a specific community.

BASIC CONCEPTS OF THE THEORY

Unitary Man—Energy Fields

Central to Rogers's model is the concept of "unitary man."[4] In this context unitary refers not only to wholeness and interconnectedness within the human person but also to the interconnectedness of the human being with the universe. Rogers's view of the person and the environment reflects the perspective of relativity theory. Matter and energy are one and the same and thus interchangeable. All that there is can be conceived of as an energy field. An energy field is electrical in nature, consisting of waves of electron particles. Matter is an energy field which is manifested in dynamic wave patterns visible to the human eye. Every visible object, including the human, is also surrounded by a field consisting of wave forms whose patterns are not visible to the human eye.[5]

Comprehending this rather abstract concept is difficult. It may be helpful to consider a light bulb. A light bulb is an apparently solid object; when lit it produces both a visible field—light—and an invisible field—heat. Both heat and light are energy forms. The electron flow produced when the lamp is plugged into the electrical current converts the filament from matter to energy, that is, heat and light. Humans also take in matter and energy from their environment and produce a usually invisible field of heat and a usually invisible field of light, as demonstrated by Kirlian photography.

Why is the concept of energy fields important? What difference does it make whether man and environment are perceived as matter or as an energy field? If humans and their environment are perceived as energy fields, then all boundaries are arbitrary. Everything is connected to everything else. We are one with the universe, continually affecting and being affected by it. The universe is the ultimate open system. Humans, individually or as an aggregate—that is, a community—must be considered as wholes greater than the sum of their parts. Moreover, the human can not be considered apart from the environment. In Rogers's[6] view, environment includes all the animate and inanimate fields external to man. Because the human and environmental fields extend infinitely, simple local cause and effect can not be considered adequate to explain changes in the system. Each interaction between the human and the environmental fields produces changes in each, which in turn send a wave of changes throughout the entire system. The changes can not, however, be said to be caused by a specific event. The best that can be said is that a given event contributed to the changes. In addition, the changes in the system are not limited by the usual boundaries of space and time but, rather, operate in a four-dimensional universe of spacetime.

Spacetime—Four-Dimensionality

In everyday life we perceive the universe as three-dimensional. Space and time are separate but real boundaries to our existence. Time is a finite entity which flows like a river through our lives. Space is defined by the matter that fills it or by the apparent emptiness surrounding the matter. That an object can occupy only one space at a given point in time seems self-evident. Energy, however, is not confined by space. Humans and their environment as energy fields can occupy infinite space and overlap with the space occupied by other fields. Although the visible energy field, matter, may appear to be confined to one space at a time, consciousness, a manifestation of energy, can range freely both in space and in time.[7] An example is sitting in one's living room and imagining oneself in Hawaii at a past or future time. Although the body has not left the couch, one experiences being in Hawaii, and during the experience all sense of time is lost.

During this "imaginary" journey one has consciously entered the fourth dimension, where space and time no longer bind. Individuals who exhibit paranormal abilities, precognition, clairvoyance, and so forth are operating in the fourth dimension without conscious effort. They are able to contact the past, present, or future anywhere in the universe and to experience it. These individuals are often referred to as "sensitives," and, indeed, they are sensitive to energies beyond their immediate fields.

Traditional concepts of space and time imply separateness. The concept of spacetime, or the fourth dimension, transcends the artificial boundaries imposed by space and time, implying the interconnectedness which is an essential quality of an open universe of interacting energy fields. Spacetime also demolishes any obstacles to the resonance of change through the system.[8]

The concept of spacetime is based on the special theory of relativity. Perceptions of time and space are a function of the rate at which an object is moving relative to the observer. "The faster an object moves in relation to the observer, the slower its clock runs and the shorter it becomes."[9] When two fields are moving at the same speed, time becomes timeless and space is meaningless. If the universe is, in fact, timeless, then as our fields move into synchrony with the universe we cease to perceive time as passing. Time just is Space and, therefore, distance no longer bind us.

In attempting to comprehend this concept, the biggest pitfall seems to be that of equating field motion with body motion, brain wave motion, or other commonly used three-dimensional measures. Field motion can be measured only relative to the motion of the implicate order. Beneath the explicit order of the universe, which is seeming chaos, is an implicate order characterized by oneness, unity, and perfection.[10] When our fields are in harmony with this implicate order, we can draw upon it and channel its energies to heal our own wounds and those of our fellows. In other words, we can repattern the fields in synchrony with the underlying order of the universe.[11] Human development and human field motion thus are measured by patterns of wholeness in relation to the underlying order of the universe. Before proceeding to the concepts of pattern and organization and life processes, let us consider the implications of the notions of energy fields and of spacetime for community assessment.

Viewing humans and their environment as indivisible whole open systems in mutual simultaneous interaction with an infinite four-dimensional universe undergoing constant change results in several important implications for nurses

---

doing a community assessment. We must remember that in order to study a community we must draw artificial boundaries to isolate a manageable segment of the system. Thus, it is imperative that we assess the community's multiple interactions with both its subsystems and its suprasystems, including those which may seem far removed in space and time. In addition, we must be continually aware of the dynamic nature of the system. Change is occurring even as the community is assessed, and the very process of assessment produces changes in both the community and the individual(s) assessing the community. Lastly, the assessment data collected must reflect the wholeness of the community. Reducing the community to its parts and summing them together will not provide an accurate picture of the whole. Because most of us have been schooled to study parts rather than wholes, this task seems difficult indeed. The addition of the fourth dimension and the need to assess the synchronous interaction of human field motion and environmental field motion further complicate matters. Pattern and organization provide a means of conceptualizing wholeness in a four-dimensional universe.

Pattern

Rogers uses the concept of pattern to describe the wholeness of the human and environmental fields.[12] Patterns characterize whole fields. They are the means by which we identify a field. Upon meeting a friend we immediately recognize the person as a whole. The pattern presented is one that looks, sounds, and feels like our friend. We don't stop to consider that this must be our friend because she's a 5'4" woman with brown hair, blue eyes, a relaxed walk, and a bright smile. Rather, we perceive a pattern of energy—light, sound, motion, and consciousness—that we immediately identify as our friend.

Pattern includes the structure and function of the field. Both structure and function are dynamic, but they are differentiated by the speed with which change occurs. Structure undergoes change very slowly; function changes rapidly. Structure describes the what; function, the how. Specific structural and functional characteristics differentiate the human from the environmental field.[13] The human field is characterized by the capacity for thought, feeling, creativity, and self-knowledge. These characteristics are structural elements. The interchange between these structural elements and the environment constitutes the function. Much of the descriptive data concerning the physical and demographic aspects of the community and the configuration of the formal communications networks can be categorized as structural. An example of the functional aspects of the community pattern include interaction patterns, such as high stress. Stress is a field phenomenon altering both the structure and the function of the human field. Stress is a signal of dysharmony in the human–environment interaction. Reduction of the stress requires an alteration in the human–environment interaction pattern. The change is not a passive adaptation of the human field to the environmental demands.[14] The change is an active choice to manipulate the human or the environmental field to achieve some probable outcome.

For example, I may perceive that my boss is becoming unhappy with the way I am doing my job. I feel stress, and this feeling resonates through my field. I behave differently, perhaps trying ever harder to please her. I send signals—wave patterns—verbally and nonverbally that indicate my discomfort. My time perception becomes distorted. Time may seem to race or to drag, and my body motion may reflect this distortion. These changes in my field are received by my boss, who in turn may further alter her interaction with me. If the stress response continues, it will eventually be reflected by structural changes in both fields. I have, however, a choice. I can manipulate the environment, perhaps by asking my boss what problem she perceives. I can continue to attempt to figure out what is displeasing her. I can withdraw or treat the stress symptoms with alcohol or drugs. I can meditate, bringing my field into harmony with the implicate order, decreasing my functional stress pattern as well as putting the dysharmony into perspective. My boss has the same options. I can not predict the outcome, but I can identify the probable outcomes of each course of action.

In the community, structural and functional patterns indicative of dysharmony include a high incidence of drug and/or alcohol abuse, stress-related diseases, violence, depression, and so forth. We must, however, keep in mind that these are only symptoms of dysharmony. Identification of the source of dysharmony requires that one assess the developmental life process of the community and the delays or irregularities in evolution toward its highest human capabilities.

Life Process

Life process is a crucial unifying concept within the model and provides the basis for identifying nursing problems. Life process describes the rhythmic pattern of development of the human interacting with the environment. Change is postulated to proceed in a rhythmic spiral in the direction of increased complexity and diversity of energy field patterns. Behavioral manifestations of changes in human field patterns are seen as an increasing capacity for humanness—self-knowledge, thought, and feeling. Death is a transition to a pure energy state, characterized by presumably even greater human capacities.

The patterns of development within this evolutionary process never repeat. Although some patterns may appear to be *like* previous patterns, the intervening human–environment interactions invariably produce substantive changes in the pattern.[15] At any given moment in spacetime the pattern of the human field is determined by the preceding evolution and the current interactions. Assessment of the human field and of the changes over time provides a point from which the nurse can develop probabalistic statements concerning the changes which will result from future human–environment interactions. Purely predictive statements can not be used, because all the factors contributing to change can not be specified. Probabalistic statements define what will probably happen given previous history and current activity.[16] Certain knowledge is impossible; thus interventions are based upon probable outcomes.

Rogers defines nursing's central focus as man evolving through the life process. "The aim of nursing is to assist people in achieving their maximum health potential."[17] Nurses function as an environmental force to repattern the human–environment interaction to "strengthen the coherence and integrity of the human field," and to increase the harmony of man–environment interaction.[18]

Dysharmonies in the human–environment interaction appear as delays or irregularities in the evolution of the life process. Health is a function of the evolution of the life process. Rogers does not specifically define health or illness. Both health and illness are described as value terms whose meanings vary considerably. Health is, however, one of the four concepts basic to nursing, and Rogers repeatedly uses the term.[19,20] In the context of the model, health is implicitly defined as a process resulting in a pattern of human development which will probabalistically result in increased complexity, diversity, and coherence of the human field which will in turn promote harmonious interaction with the environmental field. Operationally, optimum health is identified as a pattern of increasing human capacities—thought, feeling, and self-knowledge—paired with harmonious human–environment interactions.

As the life process is a unidirectional continuum, so health, too, is a unidirectional continuum. It is possible to get stuck somewhere along the continuum, as demonstrated by delays in the life process, but it is not possible to regress to a previous state.

From the perspective of the life process, some dysharmonies or delays which have traditionally been defined as illness are perceived as growth states which provide opportunities for the individual or group to move forward in the life process and to optimize health.

An excellent example of this is the experience of Jess Lair,[21] author of *"Ain't I a Wonder and Ain't You a Wonder Too"* and other books. Jess was an archetypical Type A person, and at age 36 he had a serious heart attack. As a result of his "illness," Jess reexamined his values, goals, and fears. He became more focused on developing his human capabilities and less concerned about his material capabilities. He changed professions; he became a psychologist and teacher as well as the author of several self-help books in which he shares his growth experience with others. From a traditional perspective, Jess was ill. From the perspective of the life processes, the "illness" actually contributed to his movement toward optimum health.

In order to assist the client to move in the direction of optimum health, the nurse must be able to identify delays in the evolution of the life process. New assessment tools that reflect the holistic, dynamic nature of the human field must be developed. Rogers proposes that delays in the evolution of the life process can be identified through the use of a series of measures she labels correlates of human development[22] (Table 19-1). These postulates are theoretical derivations from the model. Valid reliable measurement tools to test all these postulates have not yet been developed. Fitzpatrick and Donovan[23] have done substantial work on developing tools to measure perception of time passage. Their research tends to support the postulate that time is perceived as passing more quickly as

TABLE 19-1. Postulated Correlates of Unitary Human Development

CORRELATE	MOVES FROM	IN THE DIRECTION OF	
Human field motion	longer waves →	shorter waves →	seem continuous
	lower frequency →	higher frequency →	seem continuous
	longer rhythms →	shorter rhythms →	seem continuous
	slower motion →	faster motion →	seems continuous
Time experience	time drags →	time races →	timelessness
Consciousness	sleeping →	waking →	beyond waking
Life span	shorter →	longer →	eternal
Differentiation	less →	more →	transcendence
Visibility	more →	less →	ethereal
Weight experience	heavy →	light →	weightless
Creativity	pragmatic →	imaginative →	visionary

Adapted from Rogers, ME: *Postulated correlates of unitary human development.* Unpublished handout, Intercollegiate Center for Nursing Education, 1981.

we progress through the life process continuum. Ference[24] has developed some tools measuring differentiation, creativity, and human field motion. Although these measures are designed for use on individuals, adaptation for use in the community is possible as demonstrated in the example at the end of the chapter.

The concepts of energy fields, the fourth dimension, pattern and organization, and the life process describe the model's perspective of nursing, health, person, and environment. They provide the structural pattern of the model. Synthesis of these concepts into principles describing the functional pattern of the model provides direction for application of the nursing process.

Principles of Homeodynamics

Rogers has synthesized the four basic concepts into three principles which are postulated to describe, to explain, and to predict the "nature and direction of unitary human development."[25] She calls these the principles of homeodynamics. The term homeodynamics is used to imply the constancy of change throughout the life process. The principles of homeodynamics provide the nurse with a framework for client assessment. They also are the basis upon which to make probabalistic predictions concerning the outcome of current human–environmental interactions, including outcomes of nursing interventions.

The principles of homeodynamics are resonancy, integrality, and helicy.[26] The principle of resonancy states that: "the human field and the environmental field are identified by wave pattern and organization manifesting continuous change from lower-frequency, longer wave patterns to higher-frequency, shorter wave patterns."[27] The implications of this principle for nursing assessment are that the pattern of the human and environmental field as a whole needs to be assessed from the perspective of the rhythmic correlates of human development proposed in Table 19-1.

Application of the correlates to client assessment provides specific data concerning the wave patterns of the human field and their rhythmic development. Analysis of the assessment data in relation to the changes predicted by the principle of resonancy produces specific diagnostic descriptions regarding the current state of the human field. Applying the principles of integrality and helicy provides the basis for developing outcomes and interventions to alter the human field motion and thus to promote rhythmic evolution through the life process.

The principle of integrality states that "the interaction between the human and environmental fields is continuous, mutual and simultaneous."[28] This principle describes and predicts the mechanism through which changes in the wave pattern of an energy field occur. Integrality predicts that repatterning will occur whenever two or more fields interact. This principle does not assume causality. Whenever two human fields (such as the client and the nurse) interact, both will change. The interaction in and of itself is not the cause of the change or repatterning, because our interconnectedness with the universe makes it impossible to isolate any given interaction. The most we can say is that the interaction contributed to the change.

The nurse must assess the pattern of multiple human–environment interactions in relation to the current energy field pattern. From such assessment specific diagnostic statements concerning dysharmonies in human–environment interaction contributing to delays in the evolution of the life process can be developed. Interventions to alter the resonancy of the field are based upon the principle of integrality. Integrality is inherent in each step of the nursing process.

Integrality is subsumed under the third principle, helicy. The principle of helicy states that "the nature and direction of human and environmental change is continuously innovative, probabalistic, and characterized by increasing diversity of human field and environmental field pattern and organization emerging out of the continuous, mutual, simultaneous interaction between human and environmental fields and manifesting in non-repeating rhythmicities."[29] The principle of helicy provides the basis for predicting probabalistically the outcomes of current human–environment interaction as well as the desired outcomes of nursing intervention. Helicy thus provides the basis for planning and evaluating nursing interventions in relation to the life process.

Figure 19-1 represents the relationships among the principles of homeodynamics, the life process, and the nursing process. The client in this model may be a single human field or an aggregate field, such as a community. The inputs into the nursing process system are the previous life process development and the current resonancy of the unitary human fields of the nurse and the client. Assessment begins at this point. The client becomes aware of a delay or dysharmony, which impels him or her to seek help. The professional nurse's field by definition within this model includes, in addition to a unique human pattern, specific capabilities which are continually assessed. Essential components of the nurse's field include knowledge of unitary man and the nursing process, judgment, creativity, and compassion.[30]

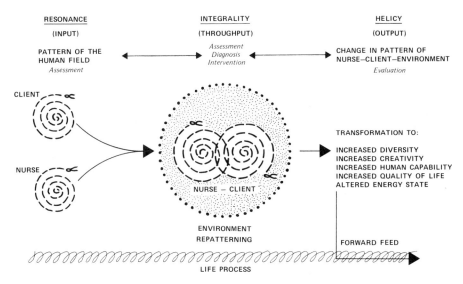

RESONANCE	INTEGRALITY	HELICY
(INPUT)	(THROUGHPUT)	(OUTPUT)
PATTERN OF THE HUMAN FIELD	*Assessment Diagnosis Intervention*	CHANGE IN PATTERN OF NURSE–CLIENT–ENVIRONMENT
Assessment		*Evaluation*

CLIENT

NURSE

NURSE – CLIENT

TRANSFORMATION TO:

INCREASED DIVERSITY
INCREASED CREATIVITY
INCREASED HUMAN CAPABILITY
INCREASED QUALITY OF LIFE
ALTERED ENERGY STATE

ENVIRONMENT
REPATTERNING

FORWARD FEED

LIFE PROCESS

FIGURE 19-1. Diagram of Rogers's model.

Assessment continues in integrality as the unitary human fields of the nurse and the client interact. Through the interaction, intervention or repatterning has already begun. Together, the nurse and the client assess and define the delay or dysharmony in the life process and the desired outcome of the nurse–client interaction. The nurse then applies his or her knowledge and skills to propose and, when indicated, to implement interventions designed to achieve the desired outcomes, which are stated in terms of increasing human capabilities.

Evaluation involves the application of the principle of helicy to determine the change in the human field pattern in relation to desired outcomes.

In order to simplify the discussion, each step in the nursing process has been described separately. It must be remembered, however, that each step is carried out continuously and that repatterning and evolution of the life process is continuously occurring.

COMMUNITY ASSESSMENT—AN EXAMPLE

Operational Definitions of Terms

Community assessment in the context of Rogers's model requires assessment of the evolution of the life process in terms of helicy, resonancy, and integrality. Operational definitions of these terms in relationship to the community are necessary. The life process of the community is the history of the community. The model directs us to analyze the community's history by identifying the rhythmicity and periodicity of change over time.

Resonancy describes the current state of the human field within the community. It refers to the structural and functional interrelationships between the parts; that is, between the different individuals and groups within the community, as well as between the immediate environment and the community.

Integrality describes the current pattern of interaction between the community of concern and the other communities or groups with which it interfaces.

The correlates of human development described in Table 19-1 provide a means for assessing the resonancy, integrality, and helicy within the community. This example will highlight assessment of differentiation. Ference defines differentiation as "greater complexity, diversity and heterogeneity."[11] In more community-specific terms, differentiation can be defined as a variety of values, life styles, ages, interaction patterns, and functions among individuals within the community and among communities within the larger context of cities, states, nations, and the universe.

Dysharmonies or delays arising from differentiation within the life process of the community may be manifested by patterns of conflict. Interpersonal, intergroup, and environmental conflict may be identified by changes in the structure and function of the field. These changes may be manifested by feelings such as tension or stress, and by behaviors such as expression of differences of opinion or values, power struggles, polarization, avoidance of one group by another, name calling, and so forth, as well as by illnesses in individual members. It must be remembered, however, that conflict or dysharmony in the context of this model does not have a negative value but is, rather, a mechanism for change and movement toward greater human capabilities. Unresolved conflict is a marker indicating a delay in the evolution of the life process as well as a means of accelerating the evolution of the life process.

APPROACH TO COMMUNITY ASSESSMENT

The descriptive approach to community assessment, discussed in Chapter 4, seems to be the method that is most consistent with Rogers's model. This approach requires that individuals performing the assessment become immersed in the total field of the community; be aware of their own knowledge, experience, and values as they relate to the community; and accept the subjectivity of experience. Rogers's model assumes that reality is defined by our perceptions. Field phenomena are communicated and received holistically. Thus subjective data assume an important role in assessment.

Epidemiological data may be incorporated later into the assessment as a means of identifying community-specific symptoms of dysharmony or factors contributing to the dysharmony. The systems approach is inherent in the analysis of data within the model.

The following example will illustrate the application of the model to a specific community.

Peaceful Valley

Peaceful Valley is a community of 500 residents within the larger community of Spokane, Washington. The visible field of Peaceful Valley is separated from the larger community field by a number of natural barriers. Peaceful Valley is bounded by high cliffs to the south and the Spokane river to the north. The cliffs and the river curve outward to form an oval-shaped bowl. The downtown shopping and business area lies above the valley only three blocks away to the east. The valley is not visible from the adjacent metropolitan area. Clarke Street, the only through street in the valley, is accessible from one of the major thoroughfares in the downtown area. To the west, Clarke Street rises out of the valley to a Y. One arm of the Y continues up to a residential area on the southern cliffs, and the other arm meanders along the river and provides access to an area approximately one mile downstream called People's Park which is used for nude sunbathing and occasional partying by the younger, less-conservative members of the greater Spokane community. Towering above the valley and casting a very large shadow is the Maple Street Toll Bridge. The bridge is a significant source of noise, especially at peak traffic hours, as well as of trash and other debris, which rain down on the valley.

Peaceful Valley is very quiet except for the noise from the city above. In spring and summer, it is lush and green. As one moves from the riverbank toward the cliffs, there are increasing numbers of tall, stately, old maple trees, and evergreens surrounded by deep undergrowth. Looking south from the riverbank, the valley rises about 500 feet, and the streets give the impression of a series of terraces. Most of the homes are small frame structures built in the early 1900s. The average house is 60 years old. The per room valuation of the houses is the lowest in the city. Many of the houses are brightly painted, with well-kept yards; others are weather-beaten or display layers of peeling paint and have yards knee-high in weeds. Nearly every house has a woodpile and a vegetable garden. Many homes also have chickens and other fowl. Most of the homes near the river's edge are occupied by renters. These residents tend to be younger persons, many of whom are artisans and craftsmen who have chosen a life style different from that of the mainstream culture. In addition, there are a number of homosexual families living in this area. As one proceeds toward the cliffs, the homes are more likely to be occupied by the owners, and the residents are older. Forty-one percent of the residents of Peaceful Valley are 62 years old or older, 41 percent are between 22 and 61 years old, the remaining 18 percent are 21 years or younger.

At the far eastern end of the valley, halfway up Clarke Street, is a small community center brightly painted with artwork done by the residents. Just below the community center is the valley's only business, a casket company employing 15 persons, none of whom live in the valley. A small community-maintained and community-supported park is located beneath the pylons of the Maple Street Bridge. An elderly brick school building, now closed and boarded up, is located in the center of the community.

Residents must leave the valley to shop and to obtain all other needed services. Access to areas outside the community is provided by city bus, a disabled person's van, private car, or by walking either up Clarke Street or up a very long set of stairs which scale the cliff to the southeast.

Although the visible field of the community is relatively isolated from the greater Spokane community, its invisible energy field is not. Nearly everyone in Spokane has heard of Peaceful Valley, though most persons have never been there. The valley has been the subject of numerous newspaper, radio, and television news stories. These news stories have influenced the way the community is perceived by nonresidents. News stories have presented the area from a historical perspective, emphasizing its continuous habitation from early Indian times, its growth as an immigrant community in the early 1900s, and its steady decline into a community populated by rugged individualists intent upon living an alternate life style—generally considered to include extensive drug use and a degree of promiscuity. Other articles have highlighted current and continuing issues between the community of Peaceful Valley and the larger Spokane community, emphasizing the solidarity of the community spirit. The issues addressed have ranged from anger concerning the noise and debris raining down upon the community from the Maple Street Bridge to attempts by the community to have the area named a national historic landmark as a means of obtaining funds for renovation of the existing housing and of preventing large-scale development within the area.

Given these data concerning the community; combined with the knowledge, values, and experience of the individuals or group processing the data; one could have a number of preconceptions concerning the community. Identifying these preconceptions and then strolling through the community and immersing oneself in the community's field will, through the aegis of integrality, result in altered perceptions. A group of students whose assignment was to assess Peaceful Valley described the changes in their perceptions as follows:

> At first our group saw this area only as a rundown, poor, isolated section of town. Upon closer observation another aspect of this area began to emerge. As its name implies, it was peaceful (very)—the river slowly rolling by, lovely trees, birds singing, flower and vegetable gardens here and there, even some livestock, a center for activities and above all a community spirit rising out from the tattered buildings.[32]

This holistic impression reflects the relationship between the community's field motion and the implicate order. The sense of calm, quiet harmony perceived by the students suggests that the community's energy field is basically in harmony with the environment but does not imply that there are no dysharmonious interactions.

Further data in relation to differentiation within the community and between the community and the surrounding environment provide specific information concerning the presence of dysharmonies in the evolution of the life process of the community and give direction for developing nursing diagnoses and interventions.

Differentiation within the Life Process of the Community

The development of differentiation within the community of Peaceful Valley over time can be illustrated using a unidirectional continuum (Fig. 19-2). Delays in development or crisis-conflict points are illustrated by small, closely spaced spirals. Slow, steady development is illustrated by more widely spaced spirals. The addition of new groups of individuals to the community with different values, cultural beliefs, and interaction patterns provides one means of identifying points along the continuum when forces favoring increased differentiation are present. Historical data concerning the community indicate that at those points at which the forces favoring increased differentiation were greatest, conflict between groups was most prominent.

Figure 19-2 illustrates the process of differentiation over time in the community of Peaceful Valley. Major population changes usually occur at 20-year intervals, but influences external to the community—such as economic depression, war, and social unrest—have obvious effects upon the periodicity of change and must be taken into account in predicting future differentiation. As Figure 19-2 illustrates, Peaceful Valley has demonstrated steady increase in differentiation since before the establishment of the city of Spokane. The community has progressed from a group of a few extended Indian families who shared the same culture, values, and interaction patterns to the present-day mix of young and old persons from a variety of cultural and social backgrounds whose values and beliefs are widely divergent. As the community developed to its current level of diversity and complexity, conflicts between community members and between the community and surrounding communities have been prominent. Past experience with successful resolution of conflict and integration of new members into the community provides a basis for probabalistic predictions

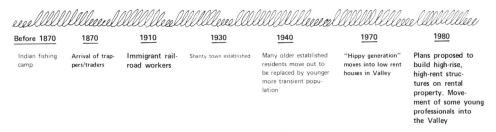

FIGURE 19-2. This unidirectional continuum illustrates the development of differentiation within the community of Peaceful Valley over time.

concerning the community's ability to resolve present and future conflicts and to proceed in the direction of ever more complexity and diversity. The current state of the community's field is a function of its past, thus the resonance of the community field must be viewed against this historical background.

Resonancy

The current state of the field reflects both unity and conflict which emerge from the high degree of differentiation within the community. In interviews with the residents, it became clear that there was a substantial amount of conflict between the older and the younger residents. This conflict seemed to contribute to the health problems identified by the residents. Concomitantly, however, there was a feeling of unity concerning their affection for the community. The older residents expressed a high degree of suspicion about the younger residents and their "strange" life styles. Visible evidence of the concerns of the elderly population are reflected in the increasing number of barrier fences and "No Trespassing" signs seen as one moves from the river toward the cliffs. Multiple locks and an unwillingness to open the door to strangers are further evidence of the fear felt by older residents. In interviews of these elderly members of the community, many expressed disdain for the "transients and hippies." The primary health problem identified by these older individuals was loneliness and isolation. Although the community center provides some social and health maintenance programs, many of the elderly residents have no car and are unable to trek uphill to the community center. Despite these problems, most of the elderly residents expressed affection for the area and said they would rather live here than anywhere else.

Most of the younger residents of the valley chose to live in Peaceful Valley in order to pursue their own values and life styles. Most expressed rejection of the materialistic values of the mainstream culture and were more concerned with self-sufficiency than with upward mobility. They admitted to problems related to low income, especially the cost of heating, but in general expressed acceptance of these problems as the price of meeting other, more important, needs. Like the elderly residents, this group expressed affection for the area and a desire to maintain the essential character of the community. The younger residents were aware of the feelings of the older residents but seemed unconcerned as long as they were left alone. The two most commonly mentioned health problems in this group were drug and alcohol abuse.

Given these data, one could state a community diagnosis as "Dysharmony between the older and younger residents related to differences in life styles, values, and interaction patterns." Specific symptoms of the dysharmony include the suspicion, loneliness, and isolation felt by the older population and the disaffection of the younger residents, which may contribute to drug and alcohol abuse.

The principle of helicy predicts that change in this situation will occur only through interaction between the two fields and that such change will result in both increased harmony and increased differentiation. Thus nursing actions need to be directed toward increasing contact between the fields of the elderly and the younger residents. Many options are available to accomplish this. Essential to the success of any intervention, however, is agreement by both groups concerning goals and means. Some possible strategies to increase contact of the visible fields might include a younger family group adopting an older family group, younger residents providing transportation for the elderly population, a community farmers' market, or perhaps a community-pride project which would encourage the sharing of skills and knowledge between the two groups. Because most of the elderly persons pray and many of the younger people meditate, increased contact between the fields transcending time and space could be accomplished by individuals or groups focusing meditative or prayful loving thoughts on the opposing group.

Mutual involvement of the two groups in dealing with a common concern provides another likely means of increasing contact between the fields. Threats to the community from outside often provide a common issue for collaboration.

Integrality

The residents of Peaceful Valley expressed a sense that "Spokane looks down upon them both physically and psychologically." Indeed, in the larger community, Peaceful Valley is viewed as a disadvantaged neighborhood populated by weirdos and hippies and is generally labeled a "bad part of town." Interestingly, the crime rate, which is often used to label communities as "bad," is no higher in Peaceful Valley than in the more affluent neighborhoods surrounding it, and crime is not perceived as a particular problem by the residents.

In addition to this prevailing attitude, over half the property in the valley is owned by absentee landlords. These landowners are well aware of the potential of this area for income-producing development. The residents of Peaceful Valley, however, are united in their desire to maintain the community in its present form. The recent addition of some young professionals to the community has provided resources for the community to make its wishes known at the city, state, and national levels. The current request to the national historic landmark commission is a tangible result of community efforts to maintain itself and to determine its future direction. This effort provides an indication of the direction in which the community wishes to move and its willingness to work through preestablished channels within the suprasystem. Such actions on the part of the community increase the awareness of the larger community concerning this area and present a view that varies from that which currently prevails. These altered perceptions in turn result in increased interaction between the community of Peaceful Valley and the surrounding community, which according to the principle of helicy, should result in increased differentiation of consciousness within both Peaceful Valley and the larger community field.

The community diagnosis related to this problem may be stated as "Dysharmony in integrality between Peaceful Valley and the larger community of Spokane related to limited interactions and disparate goals and values."

Once again the principle of helicy predicts that change will occur as interaction increases. When the community presents itself as a vital developing field, then the perceptions of the larger community will tend to be altered in this direction. In the process of projecting this image, a common goal which unites the two groups within the community can be used to increase the interaction between these groups and thus to move the community toward greater differentiation.

A variety of strategies are possible to increase interaction between the two community systems. Conflict management theory provides one basis for developing interventions to achieve this goal. Because this conflict has been long standing and unresolved, interventions to escalate the conflict paired with community efforts to publicize their position might prove fruitful in increasing the interaction and in bringing the conflict to resolution. The exchange of ideas will contribute to increasing the diversity of consciousness within and concerning the community and lead to creative solutions which improve the quality of life for both. There is no one correct intervention. Using the principles of the model and personal knowledge, experience, and creative energies, one can develop some interventions which will probably achieve the desired outcomes.

The student of today will find himself or herself working in a world of nursing where holistic interactive models of persons and nursing predominate. Rogers's model provides a paradigm for such models. Today's nursing students will develop the tools and supporting theories which are necessary to intervene to meet the needs of the whole person and to maximize health rather than to treat disease. The community is the natural arena for such holistic, health-maximizing nursing practice. Adaptations of Rogers's model to assess and to intervene in the community will provide a springboard catapulting us into that future. This chapter is designed to provide an introduction to the theory, one interpretation of the elements of the theory, and a limited example of its application. This chapter is a beginning. The readers who experiment with and further develop the model will contribute significantly to the life process of the nursing profession, which must change and evolve toward its greatest human capabilities if it is to survive as a viable human service.

REFERENCES

1. RIEHL, JP AND ROY, C: *Conceptual Models for Nursing Practice*, ed 2. Appleton-Century-Crofts, New York, 1980, p 3.

2. GEORGE, JB (ED): *Nursing Theories: The Base for Professional Nursing Practice*. Prentice-Hall, Englewood Cliffs, NJ, 1980, p 164.

3. ROGERS, M: *An Introduction to the Theoretical Basis of Nursing.* FA Davis, Philadelphia, 1970, pp 43–47.

4. ROGERS, M: *Nursing: A science of unitary man.* In RIEHL, JP AND ROY, SR. C (EDS): *Conceptual Models for Nursing Practice,* ed 2. Appleton-Century-Crofts, New York, 1980, p 330.

5. ROGERS, op cit, p 62.

6. Ibid, pp 49–54.

7. DOSSEY, L: *Space, Time and Medicine.* Shambala, Boulder, CO, 1982, p 142.

8. Ibid, p 143.

9. WOLF, A: *Taking the Quantum Leap: The New Physics for Non-Scientists.* Harper & Row, San Francisco, 1981, p 182.

10. DOSSEY, op cit, pp 181–189.

11. WEBER, R: *Philosophical foundations and frameworks for healing.* Revision Journal, Fall 1979.

12. ROGERS, 1970, op cit, pp 61–65.

13. Ibid, p 62.

14. Ibid, p 50.

15. Ibid, p 55.

16. MUTH, S AND RANK, J: *Martha Rogers's model.* In FITZPATRICK, J AND WHALL, A: *Conceptual Models of Nursing: Analysis and Application.* RJ Brady, Bowie, MD, 1983, p 254.

17. ROGERS, 1970, op cit, p 86.

18. Ibid, p 122.

19. Ibid, p 333.

20. ROGERS, 1980, op cit, p 331.

21. LAIR, J: *Ain't I a Wonder and Ain't You a Wonder Too!* Doubleday, Garden City, NY, 1977.

22. ROGERS, M: *Postulated correlates of unitary human development.* Unpublished lecture notes, Intercollegiate Center for Nursing Education, 1981.

23. FITZPATRICK, J AND DONOVAN, M: *Temporal experience and motor behavior among the aging.* Res Nurs Health 1:60, 1978.

24. FERENCE, H: *The relationship of time experience, creativity traits, differentiation and human field motion.* Unpublished doctoral dissertation, New York University, 1979.

25. ROGERS, 1970, op cit, p 96.

26. KATCH, M: *A negentropic view of the aged.* Journal of Gerontological Nursing 9(12):658, 1983.

27. ROGERS, 1970, op cit, p 333.

28. Ibid.
29. Ibid.
30. ROGERS, 1970, op cit, p 122.
31. FERENCE, op cit, p 23.
32. WURZBERG, S: Unpublished community assessment report, Intercollegiate Center for Nursing Education, 1983.

INDEX

An *italic* number indicates a figure. A "t" indicates a table.